CARING FOR ELDERLY
PEOPLE

NURSES' AIDS SERIES

$$\boxed{\text{NAS}}$$

CARING FOR ELDERLY PEOPLE

Roger Watson

BSc, PhD, RGN, CBiol, MIBiol
Department of Nursing Studies
The University of Edinburgh,
Edinburgh, UK

Baillière Tindall
London Philadelphia Toronto Sydney Tokyo

| Baillière Tindall | 24–28 Oval Road, |
| W.B. Saunders | London NW1 7DX |

The Curtis Center,
Independence Square West,
Philadelphia, PA 19106–3399, USA

55 Horner Avenue,
Toronto, Ontario M8Z 4X6, Canada

Harcourt Brace Jovanovich (Australia) Pty Ltd,
32–52 Smidmore Street,
Marrickville, NSW 2204, Australia

Harcourt Brace Jovanovich Japan Inc.,
Ichibancho Central Building, 22–1 Ichibancho,
Chiyoda-ku, Tokyo 102, Japan

© 1993 Baillière Tindall

ISBN 0 7020 1587-3

A catalogue record for this book is available from the British Library.

Typeset by Photo·graphics, Honiton, Devon
Printed in England by Clays Ltd, St Ives plc

Contents

Section IV: Issues and Trends

Preface

More people are living longer and the proportion of older people in our society has grown throughout this century. While this is surely a cause for celebration it has brought with it an absolute increase in the number of frail elderly people and an increased need for health and related workers who are dedicated to their care. *Caring for Elderly People* has been written as an introduction to the relevant gerontological issues, the organizational framework and specific aspects of the nursing care of older people for student nurses and other care workers in training.

As author of this first edition I am indebted to Alison Storrs for the three editions of *Geriatric Nursing* which set the standard for books at this particular level. This first edition of *Caring for Elderly People*, however, approaches the material under four distinct headings of Ageing and Health, Care of the Elderly Settings, Aspects of Care and Issues and Trends and approaches the subject through the 'four giants'—immobility, instability, incontinence and mental impairment—which were favoured by Isaacs. The text contains only one table and one figure, but there are many boxes which summarize the key points of the chapters. References are only given where absolutely necessary and, in common with the annotated bibliography, the material cited is recent, relevant and research based.

The aim of the section on Ageing and Health is to present ageing in its present context in addition to outlining the problems which can accompany old age. Confusion in elderly people merits its own chapter due to the increasing prevalence of dementia and the fact that elderly people with dementia are cared for in a number of different settings. The importance of community care is stressed in Chapter 4 and the chapters covering assessment and rehabilitation emphasize the relationship between these two areas of care. Several of the tools used by the multidisciplinary team in the assessment and rehabilitation of elderly people are presented because nurses will increasingly be expected to understand the basis on which assessment is made and on how the success of rehabilitation is measured. Chapters 8 and 9 from the section on Aspects of Care are directly related to the concept of the 'four giants'. Chapter 10 on nutrition has been written with an increasing awareness of the adverse effects of hospital admission on nutritional status, particularly with elderly people in mind. Issues and Trends covers several controversial areas in the care of elderly people such as restraint, euthanasia and consent.

I am grateful to the publishers for the ease with which the process of writing this book, from my original ideas to publication, has gone. The work is dedicated to the patients and staff, past, present and future, of Kirklandside Hospital, Kilmarnock in Ayrshire.

SECTION I: Ageing and Health

Chapter 1
The Effects of Ageing

Caring for older people provides one of the supreme challenges of nursing and much of the work that is carried out in this area—in practice, research and education—represents all that is best about the profession. The nurse is in a unique position when working with older people to influence the outcome of care, not only through the application of sound 'hands on' practice, but in exercising skills whereby a range of other disciplines is coordinated towards a satisfactory outcome for individual elderly people.

'Care of the elderly' is one of the many areas within nursing in which nurses can specialize, thereby working exclusively with older people. This is reflected in the specialist courses run by the respective English and Scottish National Boards for Nursing, and also in the setting up within the United Kingdom professional body for nurses—the Royal College of Nursing—of the Association for Care of the Elderly (ACE). Nevertheless, it is a reasonable proposition that all nurses should have a good understanding of how to care for older people, because there are many environments in which they will be encountered. Wherever older people are being cared for—whether on a ward dedicated to care of the elderly (where they will be admitted by a geriatrician), a medical or surgical ward or in the community—they will have unique needs which call for special skills in order to deliver adequate nursing care.

The proportion of older people with whom the nurse comes into contact professionally is not representative of the whole elderly population. Most elderly people are living independently and, if ageing is causing problems, can compensate by themselves or manage, with minimal assistance, in the community. In a health-care environment, be it hospital or home, the nurse encounters a wide variety of problems in older clients, all of which can vary in severity.

Specialized Skills

The nurse working in care of the elderly has to exercise a wide range of skills. Often it is the case, with the multiple pathology frequently observed, that a range of skills will be necessary with one patient. These skills can include communication with a severely depressed or cognitively impaired person or they may involve making allowances for a person's poor vision or hearing. Good observational skills are required to monitor the progress of a hypothermic patient who is recovering, and these must be exercised in parallel with clinical skills that enable rehydration and appropriate raising of body temperature. Nutritional problems are not uncommon at home and in hospital, and considerable patience is required in helping patients who are unable to feed themselves (see Chapter 10). Some physical strength and a great deal of knowledge of lifting and transferring techniques are needed in order to help patients to mobilize safely, to prevent skin breakdown from prolonged pressure (see Chapter 9) and for help with using the toilet if incontinence is to be avoided in patients who cannot otherwise use facilities on their own (see Chapter 8).

Ageing

Ageing is an inevitable consequence of survival and the science of ageing, gerontology (literally the study of ageing), seeks to clarify the causes and the consequences of ageing. The related medical specialty of geriatric medicine seeks to understand the diseases associated with ageing and to treat them accordingly. The knowledge gained from these studies contributes towards an understanding of ageing which is embodied in the concept of 'the ageing process'. While it is true, therefore, to say that there is an ageing process and that this process is entirely normal, it is clear that this process becomes more of a burden for some than for others. It is not entirely established why some individuals suffer more from the effects of ageing than others, but some factors may be the different diseases encountered throughout life, the different occupations which people follow and, of course, the different social and economic circumstances under which people live. The process has social, biological and psychological consequences, and it is necessary for the nurse who is going to work with older people to understand something about both the normal and the abnormal aspects of ageing.

BIOLOGICAL ASPECTS OF AGEING

Biological growth and development continue until about the mid-twenties in the majority of people. From a purely biological perspective, therefore, the ageing process could be viewed as beginning at about the age when many young people are setting out on their careers with the prospect of many productive decades in front of them. Clearly the biological view of ageing has to be qualified, and an explanation of how the process of biological ageing leaves some people relatively unscathed while others are reduced to a high degree of physical dependency is required. For a summary of the biological theories of ageing, see Box 1.1.

Cellular Theories of Ageing

Biological ageing begins slowly; has more effect on some body systems than on others and accelerates in the later years of life. The underlying reasons have been the subject of much research over the past few

---

The biological theories of ageing

Cellular theories
Cells are programmed to divide only a limited number of times

Protein synthesis
With ageing, the proteins of the body—principally collagen and elastin—become less flexible and less elastic

Oxygen toxicity
As the body ages it is less able to defend itself against the toxic effects of oxygen

Immune system
Declining competence with age may lead to increased infection, autoimmune disease and cancer

---

Box 1.1

decades but a comprehensive explanation is not yet available. Theories revolve around the cell—its part in the ageing process and the consequences thereof. It would appear that cells can only divide a certain number of times; most body cells are 'programmed' to divide about 50 times. If a cell is removed from the body and grown independently in a laboratory it is observed, quite simply, that the older the subject, the fewer times the cell will divide (Spence & Mason, 1992). This gives some insight into the biological process of ageing. It shows that the potential for further cell division, which is necessary for growth and repair of tissues, diminishes with age.

In some systems, such as the nervous system, the musculature and the heart, the cells which comprise the tissues and organs cannot be replaced once they are removed by death or damage. These systems are, therefore, much more susceptible to the process of ageing, having little or no capacity for growth and repair. Obviously, as we go through life we are liable to incur more cell damage, from many sources, and this will lead to widespread cell death, with severe consequences for systems in which cells cannot be replaced.

Collagen and Elastin in Ageing

It is also observed that tissues such as skin and cartilage lose their elasticity with age, and this is related to the chemical changes in the protein components of these tissues. With age, some of these proteins (collagen in the case of cartilage, and elastin in the case of skin) are made by the body in forms that are structurally different from the corresponding proteins in the younger person. For example, more collagen that is less flexible is laid down in cartilage and the elastin in skin becomes thicker with age (Tortora & Anagnostakos, 1990a). This can easily be related to the changing appearance of the skin, which becomes less elastic and wrinkled, with age and also the decreasing mobility and speed of the musculoskeletal system.

Oxygen Toxicity and Ageing

Another theory takes into account the decreasing ability of the cells in the body to defend themselves against oxygen, which, without certain defence mechanisms, is actually a highly toxic substance. This inability to defend against toxic oxygen leads to changes in the structure of cell membranes, making them more rigid, and it also leads to genetic errors (Tortora & Anagnostakos, 1990a). The cell membrane is the means whereby cells communicate with their environment and also control that environment through the uptake of nutrients and excretion of toxic substances. The functions of the protein component of cell membranes, which are vital for the above processes, is influenced by the rigidity of the membrane. The consequence of genetic errors is poor cell reproduction by mitosis, with decreasingly efficient daughter cells in all tissues and organs. This could lead to increasing failure of body systems.

The Immune System and Ageing

That the competence of the immune system declines with ageing is established. However, the decline in competence of this system, composed of the lymphatic system and a host of specialized white blood cells, may also be a contributory factor in the ageing process.

This could be manifested in increasing infections, autoimmune disease (whereby the immune system literally begins to attack the body) and cancer.

Whatever theory or combination of theories for biological ageing is correct, the outcome of ageing, in purely biological terms, is clear. There is a progressive change in the body's ability to undergo adaptive responses (homeostasis), with a concomitant decline in function and a lowered capacity to adapt to biological stress. Such stress could include dehydration, hypothermia and disease processes (both chronic and acute).

Ageing of Body Systems

It is useful to look at a few of the systems of the body in order to see how they change with ageing (see Box 1.2). Some caution is required, nevertheless, as it is essential to differentiate between normal (i.e. physiological) ageing and those disease (i.e. pathological) conditions which are associated with ageing. One of the pitfalls which must be avoided in working with the older people is the ascribing of each sign and symptom to the process of ageing as such. It must also be appreciated that most of the work on normal ageing is done in hospitals and therefore on people who have some underlying pathological condition.

Two general points should be appreciated with reference to the decreased ability of older people to adapt to environmental changes. One is that total body water reduces with age, thereby making the elderly person increasingly susceptible to dehydration. In parallel, there is a decreasing ability to sense heat and cold and a reduction in ability to conserve body heat,

---

The physiological effects of ageing

Musculoskeletal system
Muscular atrophy, bone decalcification and postural changes

Cardiopulmonary changes
Blood vessels lose elasticity, increase in pulse rate and blood pressure

Calcium redistribution leading to decalcified ribs and calcified costal cartilage; these changes and postural changes lead to decrease in efficiency of lungs

Urinary system
Loss of diurnal rhythm of urine production and decrease in kidney filtration

Digestive system
No significant changes

Nervous system
Decline of hearing and vision

Endocrine system
Decline in gonadal function

Box 1.2

and this means that older people are more prone to hypothermia. These two aspects of ageing are very important for the nurse to understand, as they have obvious clinical significance. The elderly person who is ill will be at even greater risk of dehydration and hypothermia.

Skin and Musculoskeletal System Changes

Turning to individual systems, the changes in the skin have been mentioned earlier and the outcome of these changes is that the skin of the elderly person is very prone to damage and requires careful handling by nursing staff (see Chapter 9). The musculoskeletal system undergoes changes both in the musculature, which progressively wastes (atrophies), and the skeleton, which undergoes a progressive loss of calcium (decalcification), its main structural component (Tortora & Anagnostakos, 1990b). The latter change makes the bones of older people more prone to fracture and, again, these require careful handling by nursing staff. The decreasing elasticity of joints, due to changes in collagen synthesis, mean that these, too, are more prone to damage.

Cardiopulmonary Changes

The cardiovascular system undergoes change such that the arteries lose their elasticity. This can lead to an increase in pulse rate and systolic blood pressure (Tortora & Anagnostakos, 1990a). A change in blood pressure without any associated pathology is probably quite normal in ageing. In the respiratory system a redistribution of calcium takes place such that the ribs lose calcium and the costal cartilage gains calcium. This, in conjunction with postural changes, leads to decreasing efficiency of lung ventilation with age. For this reason, one of the worst things an elderly person can do is to have prolonged periods in bed (see Chapter 2); the changes in the respiratory system make the elderly person more susceptible to the respiratory complications of bed-rest such as chest infection, which is associated with poor lung ventilation.

Digestion and Metabolism

While minor changes in the digestive system do take place, such as decreased saliva production, it is hard to point any real decline in function. Nurses should note, particularly, that constipation is not a normal part of the ageing process. One of the accessory organs of digestion, the liver, does undergo changes: it reduces in size and its blood supply, from the digestive system, decreases. Normally this is of no real consequence but it does have an adverse effect when drugs have been administered—not an infrequent occurrence in the elderly—in that drugs are poorly metabolized. This is something that the nurse most certainly needs to be aware of since there is an increased likelihood of side-effects, overdose and adverse reactions. It is not uncommon, therefore, that smaller doses of drugs are administered to older people than are given to younger people (see Chapter 12).

Urinary System

In contrast to the digestive system, the urinary system does undergo significant changes. Most of its functions decline, for example filtration rate, excretion and reabsorption by the kidneys (Tortora & Anagnostakos, 1990c). Again, this will have an effect on drug administration to older people; they are less able to excrete drugs or the products of drug metabolism. The normal pattern of urine production is lost, such that more urine is produced at night. This may necessitate frequent visits to the toilet during the night. It is also a fact that urinary incontinence increases with age (see Chapter 8).

Nervous and Endocrine Systems

The nervous system undergoes anatomical changes with age and there is a progressive atrophy of nerve fibres. It is difficult, however, to tie in these changes with definite neurological changes which are ascribable to age alone. As discussed below, it is a common misconception that elderly people lose all their mental faculties with age; in fact, there is very little evidence for this. Nevertheless, changes such as slower reaction time and reflexes do occur along with changes in the ability to maintain posture (Matteson, 1988). Most elderly people learn to adapt to such changes but, sometimes, it is the case that such changes lead to an increased frequency of falls (see Chapter 2). It is established that both hearing and vision decline with age and this must be taken into account in working with elderly people. It is not necessary to shout, however, simply to speak clearly and directly and to ensure that an elderly person has understood what you are saying.

While there is some decline in endocrine function with age, including the gonads in both male and female, this does not necessarily mean that the elderly person is sexually inactive (see Chapter 12).

Another aspect of ageing, which has already been considered earlier, is that there is a decreased ability to fight infection. This feature of ageing has many contributory factors and will be considered in more detail in the chapter on *The Problems of Old Age* (Chapter 2).

It is the responsibility of the nurse who works with older people, whether it is in a general medical or surgical situation or in care of the elderly, to understand the potential outcomes of the 'ageing process' and to relate these to practice. An ability to differentiate as far as possible, for each individual elderly person requiring nursing care, between what is deteriorating as a result of normal ageing and what is deteriorating as a result of disease and resulting disability can only contribute to the care and therapy administered.

PSYCHOLOGICAL ASPECTS OF AGEING

The psychology of human ageing is not as straightforward as it might seem at first. The common misconception about older people is that they have a reduced capacity both in terms of memory and mental agility. However, research into the cognitive and memory abilities of the elderly as a group, and into their ability to solve problems, does not really support this picture. It is true that some elderly people may have different ways of solving problems and, in fact, under some conditions they perform better, but there is little evidence for widespread or substantial mental deterioration.

Personality, Intelligence and Attitude

Despite the difficulties in defining and measuring personality, this is thought to change little with age. Intelligence testing, which is not without its own controversies, does appear to demonstrate a decrease in intelligence with age (Cockburn & Smith, 1991). It is not clear how significant this is, and there may be no real effect on the life of an elderly person as a result of it. The attitudes of elderly people certainly differ and often conflict with those of the younger generation. It would appear that, while attitudes are often strongly held by all age groups, it is the case that attitudes in the elderly, considered as a group, are more stable and less likely to change. One thing in which elderly people are known to differ from younger people is in their attitude towards death. It has been shown that elderly people tend not to be so frightened of the concept and the reality of death. This may be an adaptive feature of ageing (see Chapter 11).

Theories of Activity and Disengagement

What is evident, nevertheless, is that the older people undergo psychological processes of which some are unique to their age group and some common to all age groups (e.g. bereavement) but undergone more frequently in older people. The process of ageing is normal but, in terms of human existence, it requires adjustment to the changes which it inevitably entails. Theories of adjustment have evolved, and two of these theories take opposing stances on how older people adjust to the ageing process in society (see Box 1.3). The disengagement theory supports the view that the

---

The psychological theories of ageing

Theory of disengagement
Elderly people gradually undertake fewer activities and there is a mutual withdrawal from society

Theory of activity
As a person ages they give up certain former activities and compensate by taking on new activities

---

Box 1.3

elderly adjust by a process of gradually and deliberately disengaging from society whilst a mutual process of disengagement by society ensues. On the other hand, the activity theory supports the view that, while certainly disengaging in a sense from certain activities, older people gradually occupy themselves with other activities to compensate and thereby find fulfilment. It is hard to reconcile these two theories, albeit that there is evidence to support both. However, evidence supporting the disengagement theory may be that it is an accurate description of what often takes place, while the activity theory describes what the elderly might do, when given the opportunity. The activity theory is very much 'in vogue' and is promoted within the health and social services. However the truth, as described by Robbins (1991), is that practice often reflects the disengagement theory.

Ageism

Whatever changes older people may undergo as they age and however these appears to those who are younger, there is a phenomenon of persistent stereotyping and discrimination which most elderly people suffer from at some time. This has been described as 'ageism' to match the other '-isms' of race and sex. The importance of this phenomenon, demonstrable in many different groups of younger people, is that the elderly are not objectively assessed as individuals for their abilities and potential. On the contrary they are, quite frankly, discriminated against on the grounds that their opinions have little value, that their faculties, both physical and mental, have deteriorated, and that they have become a burden to the society in which they live. This is most definitely a modern and a distinctly Western phenomenon (see Chapter 13). Undoubtedly, negative attitudes are held towards older people because those who are younger hold negative attitudes towards ageing and, in particular, their own ageing. This attitude, which concentrates merely on chronological ageing, demonstrates a very narrow view of ageing. Elderly people will often say that, despite some obvious handicaps or infirmities, they do not actually feel any different from how they felt in their younger days. In many cases, they are more content with life; the stresses of working life and bringing up a family have gone and they are now able to devote time to their own interests. In fact, as they have aged, many elderly people have become the people they were meant to be and the nurse certainly has a key role to play in helping this process of self-fulfilment.

The recurrent theme in research into the psychology and sociology of the older person is that there is an almost infinite variety of experience and practice amongst elderly people. This supports the view that, in common with people in every age group, each elderly person is an individual with an individual history, individual ability and individual potential for further activity. It is in this aspect of the psychology of ageing that nursing practice should be rooted.

As with the biological theories of ageing, the nurse can gain an insight into aspects of ageing through a knowledge of the psychological theories and the sociology of ageing. Nursing practice, however, should not be hinged to any particular theory of ageing. Rather, the nurse who works with older people should be aiming to help individuals to reach their own potential without forcing them to be involved in activities that are above their level of ability.

THE OUTCOME OF AGEING

While ageing has been described here as a process and reduced to two main components, the biological and the psychological, it is necessary to see how the outcome of these components, combined with the attitude of many in society towards the elderly, can influence the quality of life of elderly people. It must be appreciated that the majority of elderly people lead very active and independent lives. Moreover, they are loved and respected by their families, both in illness and in health, and their contribution to the communities in which they live is valued and acknowledged.

Deterioration

For some elderly people, however, the ageing process becomes a burden. They lose their independence both physically, for example through immobility, and even psychologically, through depression or cognitive impairment. Their physical and mental decline may be compounded by poverty, rejection by friends and family and an inability to negotiate the state system of benefits and health care.

The requirement for nursing care, either in the community or at home, may come about suddenly, as in the case of the elderly person who falls and fractures a hip or who is found at home with hypothermia. The decreased mobility which may follow a hip operation may require changes in lifestyle, and the fact that someone has suffered a period of hypothermia may bring to light the existence of problems which were previously unknown.

On the other hand, a typical pattern for someone whose contact with the nursing profession may take place gradually would be that of the elderly person with dementia (see Chapter 3). Initially the relatives, perhaps a spouse or children, may manage. As time and the disease progresses, however, an accumulation of problems can take place, including wandering, incontinence, aggression and lack of nutrition. These may precipitate the breakdown of normal family life and may even lead to abuse of the elderly sufferer (see Chapter 12). These are the elderly people with whom the nurse will come in contact; the role of the nurse is not only to compensate for the decline in physical and mental abilities but also to project a positive attitude and image of the elderly to society generally, and to project a positive image of caring for the elderly to their colleagues in nursing and related disciplines.

THE AGEING SOCIETY

It is well established that society is, in a very real sense, 'ageing'. This process has been taking place for as long as accurate demographic records have been kept and it is projected to continue for the foreseeable future, at least for another 50 years. By describing society as 'ageing', it is meant that the proportion of elderly people is increasing. This is occurring for two reasons. Firstly, with advances in medical science and improved social conditions leading to a declining mortality rate across the ages, more people are living longer. In conjunction with this there has been a decline in the birth rate over recent years, particularly in the developed countries, which has meant a decrease in the number and proportion of younger people. This is illustrated in Fig. 1.1, which shows how the relative numbers of people in two age groups in the United Kingdom changed between 1965 and 1985.

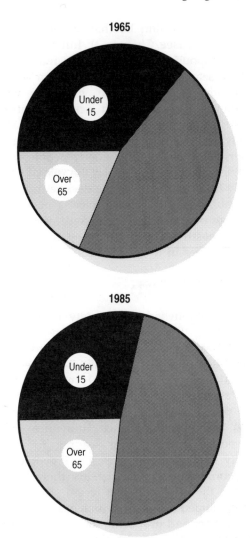

Fig. 1.1 Demographic changes in the United Kingdom: Proportion of the population comprised by two age groups. Source: Masson (1990).

Demographic Changes

The increasing proportion of elderly people in society is a worldwide phenomenon. In the 20 years between 1960 and 1980 there was a 50% increase in the number of people between 60 and 80 years of age, and this trend is continuing (Harper, 1991). In the United Kingdom there are currently 10 million pensionable elderly people and, while this proportion is not expected to increase dramatically towards the end of the century, the proportion of very old elderly, sometimes described as 'old old' (Herbert, 1992; see Box 1.4), i.e. those over 85 years of age, is expected to increase. Presently, in the United Kingdom, those over 75 years of age constitute nearly half of the elderly population and, in Europe, by the middle of the next century, 1 in 10 people will be over 75 years of age (Wolff, 1991). It is among these very old elderly that the services of the nursing profession will be concentrated.

The World Health Organization has identified the elderly as a group within society which is vulnerable to physical and mental deterioration, and it has warned that increased resources will have to be directed towards caring for them. One of the identified potential problems with having an 'ageing society' is that an economic imbalance is established whereby the ratio

---

Categorization of elderly people

Age 65–74 Young old age/elderly
Age 75–84 Middle old age/old
Age 85+ 'Old old' age/very old

Box 1.4

of older (see Chapter 13), and therefore retired, people to younger producers increases, and a smaller number of producers must support a growing population of elderly people. For example, over half of the elderly who are aged 85 years or more, it is reckoned, will require help with activities of daily living. This has to be translated into nursing and social care which has to be provided by nurses and social workers which, in turn, costs a great deal of money.

That more people are living longer and that the apparent 'normal' lifespan is also increasing should be a cause for celebration. It is a direct result of the elimination of infectious diseases such as pneumonia and tuberculosis. This has come about through the discovery and mass production of antibiotics, the introduction of immunization and much better sanitation and living conditions generally. It is necessary to educate the providers of health care and those working with the consumers, such as nurses, that the increasing proportion of elderly is a direct result of progress. This will be necessary if our attitudes towards and our provision and implementation of care are to likewise progress.

Dependency

Disability and dependency do not necessarily follow ageing. More than half of the elderly have no limits to their normal activities. Only a minority, about 5–10%, require 'hands on' care from nursing staff. Whilst appreciating, therefore, that most elderly people are healthy and independent it is necessary to focus attention, in this volume, on those who require care. Elderly people do suffer from more disabling conditions than the younger members of society and also tend to suffer from more than one chronic condition. Figures from the United States of America show that the average numbers of diagnoses rises with age. For people between 40 and 64 years, the average number of diagnoses is 2.5, whereas it is 3.1 for those aged 65–74 and 3.5 for those over 75 years. Herein lies the key to the disability suffered by a proportion of elderly people and the severe disability suffered by many of the very old elderly. From the nursing perspective, the many diseases and problems of old age converge on what have been described as the 'four giants' of geriatric medicine (Isaacs, 1981; see Box 1.5).

Four properties of the 'four giants' have been identified. Two of these relate largely to medicine and these are that they (i) have multiple problems and that (ii) there is no simple treatment. The fact that they (iii) decrease independence and also (iv) require human helpers relate largely to nursing. A discussion of how these problems arise will form the basis of the next

---

The 'four giants' of geriatric medicine

Immobility

Instability

Incontinence

Intellectual impairment

Common properties of the 'four giants'
(i)   they have multiple causes
(ii)   they destroy independence
(iii)   there is no simple treatment
(iv)   they need human helpers

Box 1.5

chapter, and the nursing care of some of the these problems will be dealt with in specific chapters later in the book.

The consequences of this increasing proportion of elderly in the population are manifold. Some diseases which are uniquely associated with ageing will increase in incidence, such as Parkinson's disease, dementia and cerebrovascular accident. In turn, this will put an ever greater strain on national budgets for health and social care. Within the health care system it will mean that an increasing proportion of resources will have to be directed towards caring for elderly people. It is already clear that there is going to be a shortage of nurses towards the end of this century, and this shortage will be felt very acutely in some areas within care of the elderly in which large numbers of staff are required (see Chapter 12).

Successful Ageing

It has been implied more than once in this chapter that the consequences of ageing are not always disability and dependence. Moreover, the research into ageing has been covered, albeit briefly, and it has been seen that research into both the physiological and the psychological aspects of ageing does not support the popular picture of mental decline and physical decay in later life. Before leaving this chapter, therefore, mention should be made of theories related to these observations and to practical implications for nursing practice and health promotion in the elderly.

Within what can be considered to be normal ageing, which is ageing without any obvious pathological condition, there have been identified two possible outcomes—either 'usual' ageing or 'successful' ageing

(Rowe & Kahn, 1987). The former is what we normally associate with ageing and the latter is what can be identified in many elderly people, i.e. ageing without serious or even significant decline in many body functions. This theory is supported by much research data. What is of interest to proponents of the theory is the identification of the different factors that dictate either usual or successful ageing. These factors have been called extrinsic factors, to distinguish them from the intrinsic biological and psychological factors which inevitably accompany ageing. Some of the issues that arise are related to the promotion of independence in the elderly. It has also been shown that good systems of social support promote successful ageing. At the biological level, there is evidence to show that moderate exercise programmes can have a significant effect on several aspects of ageing, such as loss of calcium from bones and cognitive function. Some of these will be considered in more detail later.

The relevance to nursing practice of these findings is that it is never too late to promote independence and a more healthy lifestyle in the elderly, and research is now being directed towards helping elderly people make the transition from usual to successful ageing.

CONCLUSION

In conclusion, rather than seeing elderly people as a 'burden' for society to carry, which is often how they are presented, our attitude towards the elderly generally should be that they are a resource for society, a source of stability, wisdom and guidance. Seen in this light, elderly people become a valuable asset, and they should also be valued for the contribution they have already made through the activities—commercial, educational, artistic—of a lifetime.

REFERENCES

Cockburn J & Smith PT (1991) The relative influence of intelligence and age on everyday memory. *Journal of Gerontology* **46**(1):31–36.

Harper MS (1991) Psychogeriatric Nursing. *Oasis* **7**(1):3–6.

Herbert R (1992) The normal ageing process reviewed. *International Nursing Review* **39**(3):93–96.

Isaacs B (1981) Ageing and the doctor. In Hobman D (ed.) *The Impact of Ageing*. Croom Helm, London, pp. 143–157.

Masson PR (1990) Long-term macroeconomic effects of ageing populations. *Finance and Development* **27**(2):6–9.

Matteson MA (1988) Age-related changes in the neurological system. In Matteson MA & McConnel ES (eds) *Gerontological Nursing: Concepts and Practice*. WB Saunders, Philadelphia, pp. 241–264.

Robbins SE (1991) The psychology of human ageing. In Redfern S (ed.) *Nursing Elderly People*. Churchill Livingstone, Edinburgh, pp. 19–38.

Rowe JW & Kahn RL (1987) Human ageing: usual and successful. *Science* **237**:143–149.

Spence AP & Mason EB (1992) The cell. In *Human Anatomy and Physiology*, 4th Edition. West, St Paul, pp. 58–106.

Tortora GJ & Anagnostakos NP (1990a) The cellular level of organisation. In *Principles of Anatomy and Physiology*, 6th Edition. Harper & Row, New York, pp. 53–90.

Tortora GJ & Anagnostakos NP (1990b) Skeletal Tissue. In *Principles of Anatomy and Physiology*, 6th Edition. Harper & Row, New York, pp. 141–158.

Tortora GJ & Anagnostakos NP (1990c) The Urinary System. In *Principles of Anatomy and Physiology*, 6th Edition. Harper & Row, New York, pp. 825–859.

Wolff S (1991) Wrinkles of the new age. *The Higher*, November: 15.

BIBLIOGRAPHY

Evers HK (1991) Care of the elderly sick in the UK. In Redfern SJ (ed.) *Nursing Elderly People*. Churchill Livingstone, Edinburgh, pp. 417–436.

Beginning with a look at the demography of ageing in the United Kingdom, this very interesting chapter traces the development of the care of elderly people from its origins in the poor houses to the present day.

Herbert RA (1991) The biology of human ageing. In Redfern SJ (ed.) *Nursing Elderly People*. Churchill Livingstone, Edinburgh, pp. 39–63.

Looks at ageing from the perspective of the declining ability to maintain homeostasis. Considers different systems of the body and looks at theories of ageing.

Matteson MA (1988) Biological theories of ageing. In Matteson MA & McConnell ES (eds) *Gerontological Nursing Concepts and Practice*. WB Saunders, Philadelphia, pp. 139–152.

A comprehensive, well referenced and clear look at the biological theories of ageing. This chapter comes from a section entitled Physiological Ageing Changes, *and a further nine chapters each take a detailed look at the effect of ageing on a particular body system.*

McConnel ES & Matteson MA (1988) Psychosocial ageing changes. In Matteson MA & McConnell ES (eds) *Gerontological Nursing Concepts and Practice*. WB Saunders, Philadelphia, pp. 431–480.

Approaches psychosocial ageing mostly from the social perspective. Looks in detail at the changing role of the elderly person. Mentions psychological theories of ageing.

Rice DP (1989) Demographic realities and projections of an ageing population. In Andreopolous S & Hogness JR (eds) *Health Care for an Ageing Society*. Churchill Livingstone, Edinburgh, pp. 15–46.

A very detailed look at demographic changes and many other aspects of the statistics of ageing, such as numbers of drugs taken and number of diagnoses. Mainly written from a North American perspective.

Robbins SE (1991) The psychology of human ageing. In Redfern SJ (ed) *Nursing Elderly People*. Churchill Livingstone, Edinburgh, pp. 19–38.

Very readable chapter covering the changing role of the elderly person, psychological theories of ageing and implications for the health services.

Ryan JE (1991) Building theory for gerontological nursing. In Baines EM (ed.) *Perspectives on Gerontological Nursing*. Sage, Newbury Park, pp. 29–40.

In common with all of the chapters in this book, very concise, up-to-date consideration of the issues in ageing which are relevant to nursing practice.

Shaw MW (1984) Physiological ageing. In Shaw MW (ed.) *The Challenge of Ageing*. Churchill Livingstone, Melbourne, pp. 28–35.

A very concise and informative look at the ageing of different body systems.

Chapter 2
The Problems of Old Age

In entitling this chapter *The Problems of Old Age* it should be clear to the reader, from the previous chapter, that it is not intended to convey the idea that old age is always accompanied by problems or that old age is, of itself, a problem. Rather, it is intended to give an overview of the problems, described already as the 'four giants' of geriatric medicine, which bring a proportion of elderly people into contact with nursing services. The 'four giants' help nurses to find out what the problems are with individual patients. They do not, necessarily, depend upon the presenting diagnosis of the elderly person. It is not possible to give a rundown of all the diseases that occur in geriatric medicine; these can be gleaned easily from a standard textbook of geriatric medicine. Rather, the diseases which present the greatest challenges to nursing ingenuity and demand the highest standards in nursing care will be included wherever necessary.

The 'Four Giants' of Geriatric Medicine

The 'four giants', as already given in Chapter 1 are immobility, instability, mental impairment and incontinence. The present chapter will discuss the causes and the outcomes of immobility, instability and, to some extent, incontinence. Mental impairment, due primarily to dementia, will be the subject of a separate chapter which will also look at some aspects of the nursing care of patients who are cognitively impaired (see Chapter 3). Specific chapters will be devoted to the nursing care of patients who require attention to skin care (primarily due to immobility), due to the risk of pressure-sore development (see Chapter 9), and patients who suffer from the problem of incontinence (see Chapter 8).

The 'four giants' are interesting to consider in some detail since they illustrate much about care of the elderly. All of them result from a number of different processes, related to ageing and disease, in the elderly person. Moreover, as already stated, none of them have a simple treatment or cure and all of them can lead to their own subsequent complications. They are, by no means, mutually exclusive and some severely impaired elderly people may display all four of the 'giants'. Topics relevant to this chapter, increased susceptibility to infection and disablement, are also included because, in common with the 'four giants', they have multiple causes.

IMMOBILITY

Taking immobility as an example, it is possible to draw up a list of its various causes (Box 2.1) and,

---

Causes of immobility

Physical
Fractures, pain, paralysis, exhaustion, poor feet

Psychological
Apathy, depression, confusion

Box 2.1

likewise, it is possible to list its complications. An elderly person can become immobile for both physical and psychological reasons. Among the psychological reasons could be included apathy, depression and confusion. Once immobility has become established as a result of any of these psychological factors, physical problems will ensue which will compound the immobility and lead to secondary complications.

Physical factors leading to immobility could include fractured limbs, pain on movement due to, for example, arthritis, inability to mobilize due to paralysis from cerebrovascular disease, cardiovascular disease leading to extreme exhaustion upon exertion, and feet that have not been adequately looked after. In addition, causes of immobility include the neurological, such as Parkinson's disease, in which tremor and inability to begin walking lead the subject to quite literally 'give up'. Obviously it is difficult, unless the cause is very obvious, to determine the relative influence of the physical and the psychological contributions to immobility in any individual. Immobility due to mainly physical causes will have inevitable, and detrimental, psychological consequences and vice versa. It can be seen, therefore, that whatever the primary or suspected primary cause of an individual's immobility, be it physical or psychological, a particularly vicious circle can be established whereby, without intervention, immobility can rapidly become intractable.

Complications of Immobility

Immobility brings many complications in its wake (Box 2.2). Apart from the poor psychological state, due to isolation from friends and a lack of social interaction, immobility initially leads to muscle atrophy. If the

---

Complications of immobility

Physical
Muscle atrophy, bone weakness, malnutrition,
incontinence, pressure sores, chest infection

Psychological
Isolation, apathy, depression

Box 2.2

immobility is sufficiently prolonged then the lower
limbs become useless and even contracted.
Accompanying these adverse effects on the musculature, the bones can become weakened and prone to
fracture due to progressive loss of calcium. An immobile
person for whom help is not available is inevitably
going to suffer from malnutrition and this malnutrition
is going to lead to further wastage of muscles, as
muscle protein is broken down by the body and
used to replace dietary protein. Another inevitable
complication of long-term immobility is incontinence
of both urine and faeces. If immobility leads to
bedfastness, then this will have adverse effects on the
respiratory system, whereby the individual will be
more prone to chest infection and pneumonia. Finally,
after prolonged immobility, an individual is going to
be at risk of developing pressure sores, and almost all
of the factors mentioned above will contribute towards
this.

The Multidisciplinary Team

When the nurse is presented with an immobile elderly
person it may not be obvious, at first, where to begin

with nursing care. The nurse is very quickly brought into the realm of multidisciplinary care and this care will involve both physiotherapists and occupational therapists as well as the medical staff who have made the initial diagnosis and who have responsibility for ongoing care (Box 2.3).

It will almost certainly be the case that an immobile patient will have immediate nursing requirements such as prevention of skin breakdown or management of incontinence (see Chapters 8 and 9). The course of continuing treatment and nursing care will, however, depend on what the reasons for immobility are and on how severe the immobility is. The particular strategies followed for an immobile person will be drawn up on a multidisciplinary basis, with the nurse playing the essential role of maintaining continuity of care. This may involve practical measures such as ensuring that therapy appointments are kept and

---

Members of the multidisciplinary team

General practitioner
Geriatrician
Nursing staff
  District nurse
  Health visitor
  Hospital nurse
Physiotherapist
Occupational therapist
Speech therapist
Dietitian
Chiropodist
Dentist

Box 2.3

carrying out therapeutic interventions, or less tangible measures such as motivating the patient towards desirable goals, for example greater independence. These aspects of nursing care will be covered in the chapter on *Rehabilitation* (Chapter 6).

INSTABILITY

Instability and immobility are not mutually exclusive inasmuch as many of the reasons for instability can lead to immobility. The real problem with instability is that it leads to falls and these are, unfortunately, remarkably common in older people. It is estimated that 30% of the elderly experience falls and that women fall twice as frequently as men. In some elderly people falling is a recurring problem and the number of falls increases with age. Obviously, the experience of falling, and possibly injuring oneself, for an elderly person may lead to immobility through fear of falling again or through an injury sustained due to a fall (Watson, 1992).

Intrinsic Factors

As with immobility, there are many reasons for instability and these can range from the neurological (such as Parkinson's disease) and the physiological (such as syncope) to the *iatrogenic* (resulting from medical treatment; this will be considered later in this chapter). In the latter category could be the use of prescribed drugs such as sedatives and tranquillizers. Falling, while it does appear to be linked to ageing, is not normal and it should not be accepted as part of normal ageing. Some underlying cause should be suspected and, for medical staff, the fact that an elderly person has fallen should trigger off serious investigations into the possible cause. It has been shown that, within a year of having a fall, there is an increased likelihood of dying. This is not necessarily to the fall, but to the condition which led to the fall. The fact that someone has fallen could be an indication of any of the causes shown in Box 2.4, in addition to the reasons mentioned so far. The list is by no means complete but is given to illustrate the variety of conditions which can precipitate a fall.

Extrinsic Factors

What is established about falls is that they mainly occur at home, at times of greatest activity and that, even given the above intrinsic factors, there are also extrinsic, environmental factors associated with falls (see Box 2.4). People who live alone are particularly at risk. If someone has fallen at home it will be necessary to establish what factors were involved and to minimize these for future safety. A fall does not mean that a

---

Factors leading to falls in the elderly

Intrinsic
Neurological, cardiovascular, pharmacological, cerebrovascular, malnutrition

Extrinsic
Living alone, loose rugs, trailing flexes, polished surfaces, poorly fitting carpets, poor lighting

Box 2.4

person has 'come to the end of the road' and should no longer be left alone or be incapable of looking after themselves. Features of the home, such as loose rugs, highly polished surfaces, trailing electrical flexes, badly fitting stair carpets and poor lighting, can all contribute to falls. Everything possible should be done to eliminate these features. The safety of an elderly person who has to live alone and who is prone to falls can be increased by, for example, moving to a house without stairs and installing handrails at points of particular risk such as the bathroom and in long corridors. A telephone which is accessible from the floor or an alarm system can also be installed.

Falls in Hospital

Being in an institution, such as a continuing-care setting in either a hospital or a nursing home, offers no particular protection against falls and this phenomenon has received the attention of research workers. More than half of elderly people in such settings experience falls and the most common places for this to happen are bedrooms and bathrooms. These falls take place when patients are transferring unsupervised. There appears to be no association between falls and mental confusion or self-reported problems such as sleeplessness or dizziness, but there are significant associations between falls and medical diagnoses of a neurological nature (e.g. cerebrovascular accident) and problems such as cardiovascular conditions and disease of the airways. Another significant association with falls in institutions is medication, particularly psychotropic drugs. About 90% of such accidents involved slipping out of chairs and, while these falls do not appear to be a cause of death, it is speculated that they may hasten death.

The nurse's role with respect to the patient who has fallen is not unlike that with the immobile patient. At all costs, immobility due to the fall must be prevented. At the same time, however, it may be necessary to educate the patient towards practices that will prevent falls in the future. Both falls and immobility are associated with feet that are in poor condition and, apart from referral to a chiropodist, the nurse can do much to improve and maintain the condition of an elderly person's feet. Attention to details such as nail cutting and obtaining properly fitting shoes should not be overlooked in any patients.

INCONTINENCE

Incontinence has been described as the 'unmentionable problem' (Feneley & Blannin, 1984). Unmentionable it may be, and unpleasant for the sufferer, but it is an everyday reality of nursing the elderly and there is much to learn about it and much that can be done to alleviate its consequences. The precise nursing care of urinary incontinent patients will be the subject of Chapter 8. For the purpose of the present chapter, the term incontinence will be used to mean urinary incontinence. Faecal incontinence is much less common and is nearly always caused by constipation; the alleviation of constipation will be covered in the chapter on Nutrition (Chapter 10).

Epidemiology of Incontinence

In common with the other 'giants' the incidence of incontinence increases with age. It is also the case that

more women suffer from incontinence than men.
This is particularly true of younger women, but the
difference between the sexes is also apparent in the
elderly. In women there is a difference in the prevalence
of incontinence between women who have had no
children and those who have had up to four children
(Thomas et al, 1986). After four children the prevalence
increases again, and it can fairly be said that childbirth,
which weakens the pelvic floor muscles, is the main
reason for incontinence in women. In men, the main
cause is enlargement of the prostate gland and also
the surgical procedures required to treat this condition.

Apart from the above causes it is possible to correlate
incontinence with a number of conditions and with
certain medications. For instance, incontinence has
been significantly correlated to recurrent urinary tract
infection; it is also the case that a significant majority
of demented patients and others suffering from any
neurological condition are likely to be incontinent.
One study showed that anticonvulsant muscle relaxants
are also significantly correlated with incontinence, but
it is also suspected that the use of any sedatives or
tranquillizers may increase the incidence of incontinence (Ouslander et al, 1987). It can be seen how, if a
patient who is liable to be incontinent is taking a
sleeping tablet at night, the normal stimuli that might
wake them up in order to visit the toilet could be
overridden. This subject will be given more coverage
in the chapter on *Continence and Incontinence* (Chapter
8).

INFECTION

An increasing proneness to infection occurs with
ageing, and the reasons for this are many and varied.

Older people become increasingly prone to infections (see Chapter 1) by virtue of the ageing process, but there are other factors which conspire to compound this susceptibility (Titler & Knipper, 1991).

Elderly people are more frequently admitted to hospitals and many live in long-term hospital units or in nursing homes. In such environments there is an increased risk of infection for all individuals but the risk is, not surprisingly, increased in the elderly. Such infections, which are acquired in institutions, are called *nosocomial* infections. The particular nosocomial hospital infections to which elderly people are particularly prone in decreasing order are urinary tract, surgical wound, respiratory tract, skin and bloodstream. In nursing homes, the most common nosocomial infection is again urinary tract infection, followed by skin and respiratory tract infection. The rate of nosocomial infection is at least twice as high among elderly people (70–90 years old), and may be as much as five times as high, as it is in younger people. It has been estimated that 75% of nursing home residents at some time contract a nosocomial infection.

Causes of Increased Susceptibility to Infection

The specific, intrinsic, factors in elderly people which lead to increased susceptibility to infection include the fact that the elderly do tend to suffer from more underlying diseases (Box 2.5). While this is not a normal part of ageing, it is a fact and has to be taken into consideration. Examples of disease states that lower the capacity to fight infection include malnutrition, diabetes, cancer and neurological disorders such as dementia. Malnutrition, which itself may be the result of some other underlying disease, reduces the capacity

---

Causes of increased infection in the elderly

The ageing process (reduced primary defences)
Admission to hospital
Multiple pathology
Malnutrition
Dementia
Immobility
Antibiotic therapy

Box 2.5

of the immune system. It does this, particularly in
protein deficiency, because the immune system requires
adequate protein for synthesis of antibodies which
help to fight infection. It is also the case that the
presence of vitamins, such as vitamin C, is required
for the proper functioning of the immune system.
Diabetes increases the susceptibility to infections by
impairing the immune system, and cancer, among
many of its effects, can reduce the white blood cell
count in the blood, leading to a reduced capacity to
fight infection. In a condition such as dementia there
are many reasons for an increased likelihood of
acquiring an infection, but reduced personal hygiene,
aspiration (entry into the lungs) of food while swallowing and immobility are all contributing factors. Immobility leads to collection of respiratory secretions in
the lungs where they become infected and also to
pressure sores which can harbour pathogenic micro-
organisms.

The process of ageing has an adverse influence on
several systems which conspire to increase susceptibility to infection in older people. Primary defences

such as the skin, the secretions of mucosal surfaces and the action of cilia in the respiratory tract are all impaired. Similarly, it is established that secondary defences, including cell mediated and humoral immunity, are impaired. The protective mechanism in the gastrointestinal system, which relies on commensal bacteria to give protection against pathogens, is not impaired with ageing but frequent use of antibiotics, which is common in the elderly as a group, may kill off the natural fauna of the gastrointestinal system and leave them more prone to infection by pathogenic organisms.

Prevention of Infection

An increased susceptibility to infection is something that nurses must be aware of in working with elderly people. Often it is simply a case of educating elderly people to be more aware of their own increasing vulnerability and to point out potential sources of infection, for example, around the home. In hospital, however, great vigilance and high standards of practice in the area of infection control are required if the admission to hospital is not to become a greater danger to the elderly person through nosocomial infection than the condition which necessitated admission. In practical terms this means paying attention to hand-washing procedures, as the hands are a major means of transmitting infection, and the use of disposable and even sterile disposable gloves wherever it is appropriate (Larson, 1989).

The greatest risk to the elderly person in institutional care is urinary tract infection, and this risk is greatly increased through use of indwelling catheters (Mulhall et al, 1988). Attention to fluid intake in order to encourage dilution of urine and regular voiding rather than stasis in the urinary system, combined with strict procedures to prevent cross infection when handling indwelling urethral catheters, are required.

The nurse in care of the elderly, no less than in any other area of nursing, should establish a good relationship with the area nurse responsible for infection control and should also be paying due attention to the handling of food and disposal of waste within their own area of responsibility.

DISABILITY

Finally we will look at the concept of disablement. While the 'four giants' are one way of considering the problems of old age, and nurses need to be aware of them as existing and as potential problems in every elderly person in care, they do not adequately describe the response of the individual to the ageing process. This can better be described by disablement, and this helps the nurse and other members of the multidisciplinary team (e.g. physiotherapists and occupational therapists) to evaluate how individual elderly people can carry out activities of daily living (e.g. eating, eliminating and communicating) and instrumental activities of daily living such as shopping and preparation of food.

To this end, the World Health Organization (1980) classifications of *impairment, disability* and *handicap* are worth referring to (see Box 2.6). Needless to say, there is considerable overlap between the definitions of disability but it can be seen that handicap is more severe than impairment, and that it will be easier to intervene and help the person who is impaired rather

---

Impairment, disability and handicap

Impairment
Any loss or abnormality of psychological, physiological or anatomical structure or function

Disability
Any restriction or lack (resulting from impairment) of ability to perform an activity in the manner or within the range considered normal for a human being

Handicap
A disadvantage for a given individual, resulting from impairment or a disability, that limits or prevents the fulfilment of a role that is normal (depending on age, sex, and social and cultural factors) for that individual

---

Box 2.6

than handicapped. In order to evaluate precisely the extent of disablement in an individual a process of assessment has to be carried out, and this process, which involves a well defined team of professionals and which relies on a number of standard assessment tools, will be the subject of subsequent chapters on *Assessment* and *Rehabilitation* (Chapters 5 and 6). The latter chapter, as the title suggests will consider the process of rehabilitation and the role of the nurse in this process. Rehabilitation has an outcome which is the restoration, whole or partial, of normal function. In some cases this is not possible and even partial restoration of function will still leave the elderly person with significant inability to carry out activities of daily living. In such cases the person may require *Continuing Care*, which will be covered in Chapter 7.

Factors Leading to Disability

A number of chronic conditions are predictors of disability in the elderly and these include cardiovascular disease, neurological disease and cancer (Jette et al, 1990). Other factors such as smoking and obesity are also predictors, but impaired sight and vision do not necessarily lead to disability. The process whereby chronic disease leads to disability has been studied and it appears that specific musculoskeletal decrements are important causes. Disability in terms of basic activities of daily living, such as washing and dressing, significantly ensues on impairment of the upper limbs, especially of hand function, whereas disability in terms of instrumental activities of daily living (e.g. preparing meals) is related to lower-limb impairment.

Iatrogenesis and Disability

The term iatrogenesis (literally 'caused by the physician') has been used in this chapter and in several places there have been examples of detrimental conditions which arise as a result of the admission of elderly people into hospital. Such iatrogenic disease is a major consideration in all people requiring medical and nursing care, and its severity in older people, particularly in those admitted to hospital, sometimes leads to the question of whether an individual person would be better remaining at home if there is a risk of iatrogenic disease.

Examples of iatrogenic diseases are any adverse side-effects of drugs, urinary incontinence caused by being admitted to hospital, any infections (particularly urinary) which have been contracted as a result of admission to hospital, malnutrition in hospital and pressure sores. The list of iatrogenic diseases also includes conditions such as depression, apathy and confusion.

Rather than simply accepting the existence of such iatrogenic disease, or even simply blaming it on the physicians, nurses should be aware of it and should take action, wherever possible to prevent and alleviate it. In fact, the term 'nursigenic' has been coined (Matteson & McConnel, 1988) in order to illustrate that nurses as well as physicians can be a cause of iatrogenic disease. Throughout this book there are examples of situations where nurses can prevent iatrogenesis. For example, the prevention of cross infection from indwelling catheters, through hand-washing procedures and attention to the complications of immobility.

In addition, in the area of iatrogenic disease, the nurse also has a responsibility, as was mentioned in Chapter 1, for promoting a positive attitude towards elderly people among professional colleagues. Much could be done, in this way, to prevent and alleviate iatrogenic conditions. Less deterioration would simply be ascribed to the fact that a person was old, such as confusion, and more might be investigated, such as the possible side-effect of a drug therapy.

Lifestyle and Disability

Finally, the impact of lifestyle in the health of an older person cannot be discounted. Lifestyle may refer to the present lifestyle of an individual but may also refer to the habits of a lifetime. It is generally considered

that you take the habits of a lifetime into your old
age, and this has implications for health education
which will be discussed in a later chapter. Thus
obesity, smoking, alcohol abuse and lack of exercise
may all be contributing factors to the ill health of an
elderly person. It is important to try to establish what
the normal lifestyle of an elderly person is, and in this
way the nurse can gauge the likely effect of ill health,
disability and possibly hospital admission on the
individual.

CONCLUSION

Old age is certainly accompanied by problems for a
significant number of elderly people, and care of the
elderly is largely concerned with assessing these
problems and either compensating for them or participating in the process of helping the elderly person to
overcome them and regain a degree of independence.
The 'giants' of geriatric medicine give an overall picture
of the direction of much of the activity of nurses in
any care of the elderly setting, and an appreciation of
disability, and its effects on the activities of daily
living, shows how the ageing process can be evaluated
in individuals.

This chapter has been mainly concerned with the
physical problems of ageing, leaving descriptions of
the different care settings and the care of the incontinent
patient to be dealt with in subsequent chapters. The
next chapter will look specifically at mental impairment
and the issues surrounding this problem, the prevalence
of which is increasing in line with the increasing
proportion of elderly people in the population.

REFERENCES

Feneley RCL & Blannin JP (1984) *Incontinence: Help for an Unmentionable Problem*. Churchill Livingstone, London.

Jette AM, Branch LG & Berlin J (1990) Musculoskeletal impairments and physical disability among the aged. *Journal of Gerontology* **45**(6):M203–208.

Larson E (1989) Hand washing: it's essential—even when you use gloves. *American Journal of Nursing* **89**(7):943–941.

Matteson MA & McConnel ES (1988) Gerontological nursing in acute care settings. In Matteson MA & McConnel ES (eds) *Gerontological Nursing*. WB Saunders, Philadelphia, pp. 722–761.

Mulhall A, Chapman R & Crow R (1988) The acquisition of bacteriuria. *Nursing Times* **84**(4):61–62.

Ouslander JG, Uman G, Urman HN & Rubenstein LZ (1987) Incontinence among nursing home patients: clinical and functional correlates. *Journal of the American Geriatric Society* **35**:324–330.

Thomas TM, Plymat KR, Blannin J & Meade TW (1986) Prevalence of urinary incontinence. *British Medical Journal* **281**:1243–1245.

Titler M & Knipper J (1991) Potential for infection. In Maas M, Buckwalter KC & Hardy M (eds) *Nursing Diagnoses and Interventions for the Elderly*. Addison-Wesley, Redwood City, pp. 45–69.

Watson R (1992) Steady as you go. *Practice Nursing*, March:14–15.

World Health Organization (WHO) (1980) *International Classification of Impairments, Disabilities and Handicaps: A Manual of Classification Relating to the Consequences of Disease*. WHO, Geneva.

BIBLIOGRAPHY

Abbey JC (1991) Physiological illness in ageing. In Baines EM (ed.) *Perspectives on Gerontological Nursing*. Sage, Newbury Park, pp. 275–295.

An overview of the detrimental effects of ageing. Gives particular attention to musculoskeletal changes.

Batehup L & Squires A (1991) Mobility. In Redfern SJ (ed.) *Nursing Elderly People*. Churchill Livingstone, Edinburgh, pp. 115–146.

Has some very good photographs illustrating how to safely transfer immobile patients and how to encourage mobility.

Bowling A, Formby J & Grant K (1992) Accidents in elderly care: a randomised controlled study (Parts 1, 2 and 3). *Nursing Standard* 6:29,28–30; 30,28–31; 31,25–27.

A series of articles on research into falls in the elderly, with an extensive reference list and a good consideration of the problem. Interesting comparison between nursing homes and National Health Service Wards.

Chenitz WC, Kussman HL & Stone JT (1991) Preventing falls. In Chenitz WC, Stone JT & Salisbury SA (eds) *Clinical Gerontological Nursing*. WB Saunders, Philadelphia, pp. 309–328.

An excellent, well-referenced and comprehensive chapter on the prevention of falls.

Matteson MA (1988) Age-related changes in the musculoskeletal system. In Matteson MA & McConnell ES (eds) *Gerontological Nursing Concepts and Practice*. WB Saunders, Philadelphia, pp. 171–192.

Comprehensive look at the complications of ageing and the diseases that limit mobility. Very good background reading for this subject.

Ross JER, Watson CA, Gyldevand TA & Reinboth JA (1991) Potential for trauma: falls. In Maas M, Buckwalter KC & Hardy M (eds) *Nursing Diagnoses and Interventions for the Elderly*. Addison Wesley, Redwood City, pp. 18–31.

Looks at falls and their prevention using the North American Nursing Diagnoses System. The chapter by Titler & Knipper in this volume is very good on the increased risk of infection in the elderly.

Saunder P (1989) *The A–Z of Disability.* Crowood Press, Romsbury.

Written for disabled people and using the WHO classifications of disability this is a clear, alphabetical guide to the types of disability and the equipment and organizations which are available to help.

Shaw MW (1984) Common problems of ageing. In Shaw MW (ed.) *The Challenge of Ageing.* Churchill Livingstone, Melbourne, pp. 36–45.

Poor mobility, falls and reduced functional independence are covered.

Stone JT & Chenitz WC (1991) The problem of falls. In Chenitz WC, Stone JT & Salisbury SA (eds) *Clinical Gerontological Nursing.* WB Saunders, Philadelphia, 291–308.

A good look at the aetiological factors.

Chapter 3
Confusion in Older People

The facts that elderly people form the largest single group in psychiatric care in the United Kingdom and that a great many elderly who are in continuing care suffer from mental impairment, but which is not necessarily psychiatric, lead to the conclusion that mental disorders increase with ageing. This chapter will look at some aspects of the dementias. From the nursing perspective, regardless of the precise diagnosis, it is the outcomes of the dementias which have to be coped with. Principally, confusion is the main problem but this, of course, has consequences for all of the activities of daily living.

Recent figures for the prevalence of dementia have been obtained in Scotland, which has a population of less than 10 million people. There are estimated to be 93 000 sufferers of dementia, of which 49 000 are severely demented. More than half of those with dementia are over 80 years of age, but there are about 2000 sufferers aged between 40 and 65 years. The majority of dementia sufferers live at home (80%), and of the 20% in care about half live in residential homes and half in hospital. The largest burden, therefore, in the care of demented patients, falls on the community (Killeen, 1991).

Managing confused patients requires very special nursing skills and personal qualities from the nurses who are delivering the care. The confused person may be unable to feed, may be unable to maintain continence and may even display aggression. Obviously, skills are required to compensate for these inabilities and also to generally maintain a safe living environment for the patient. Personal qualities, especially patience and consistency, are needed to deliver routine care that may have to be delivered under very difficult circumstances.

ACUTE CONFUSION

A confused elderly person may come into contact with the caring services in any number of ways—hospital admission, via the police (e.g. for wandering and being a danger to themselves), through social workers and via district nurses. Whatever the route of admission, it is essential for the medical staff to determine as quickly as possible whether the confusion is acute or chronic. By acute confusion, it is meant that the episode of confusion has had a rapid onset for some reason that is usually identifiable and that this kind of confusion is reversible. Chronic confusion, as the name suggests, has been established for quite a long time, has had a slow onset and, while some of the problems can be alleviated, is not generally reversible. The investigations which would be carried out by the medical staff would include a thorough history of the patient and the condition from a relative or other significant person, followed by complete medical examination, including blood specimens for measurement of urea levels and electrolytes and also for bacteriological culture. Urine specimens would be taken to see if any infection was present and other possible conditions such as metabolic disorders (e.g. diabetes) might be investigated. The possibility of drug or alcohol misuse would not be discounted and nutritional factors such as vitamin deficiency and dehydration would also be considered (Eccles & Wattis, 1988).

Causes of Confusion

Possible causes of acute confusion are shown in Box
3.1. Obviously, if the cause of acute confusion is
established, then a prescribed course of medical treatment will ensue in order to correct the underlying
problem and reverse the confusion. In the case of a
patient who is confused merely as a result of being
moved from familiar to unfamiliar surroundings, such
as the elderly person who has been admitted to hospital
after falling and being injured at home, the task of
reversing the confusion rests primarily with nursing
staff. It is worth bearing this in mind with all patients
and making sure that they are quickly oriented to their
new surroundings in hospital, given clear explanations
of as much as possible of what is going on around
them and made to feel 'at home' despite the fact that
they are not at home. In the case of any other patients
who are acutely confused, for whom the cause has
been established and who are undergoing treatment,
it is the responsibility of nursing staff to re-orient
them as the confusion resolves and to make sure that

Causes of confusion

Infection
Cerebral anoxia and hypoxia
Metabolic disorders
Nutritional deficiencies
Dehydration
Drugs and alcohol
Constipation
Unfamiliar surroundings

Box 3.1

confusion arising for some organic reason is not compounded by confusion resulting from a realization by the person that they are in unfamiliar surroundings.

DEMENTIA

Dementia is chronic confusion and in all the dementias there is a progressive global loss of cognitive ability with associated physical problems and there are many reasons for the occurrence of dementia (Box 3.2). The most common cause of dementia is Alzheimer's disease, in which the appearance of the brain, both superficially and microscopically, changes due to degeneration of brain cells, principally in the temporal lobes. The next most common cause of dementia is cerebrovascular disease leading to multi-infarct dementia. These two types of dementia differ in their presentation. Alzheimer's disease has a slow onset compared with multi-

---

Causes of dementia

Alzheimer's disease
Multi-infarct cerebrovascular disease
Leuwy bodies
Korsakoff's psychosis
Multiple sclerosis
Lymphoma
Herpes simplex virus
Pick's disease
Huntington's chorea
AIDS
Creutzfeldt–Jakob disease

Box 3.2

infarct dementia and there is gradual but progressive decline in cognitive ability, with no respite or improvement. On the other hand, multi-infarct dementia has a more rapid onset and tends to have a less progressive nature, rather, the sufferer will undergo discrete episodes of decline when periods of infarction occur (Thomas, 1990).

Leuwy body dementia is proving to be more common than was originally thought and is characterized by the formation of particular areas of devastation in the brain (Leuwy bodies). There are many other dementias, for example, Pick's disease, Creutzfeldt–Jakob disease and now AIDS (acquired immune deficiency syndrome) associated dementia (Mackay, 1991). All have their own characteristics either histological or, in some cases, infective organisms. From the nursing perspective, the most commonly encountered dementias are Alzheimer's disease and multi-infarct dementias. These do have slightly different characteristics, as outlined above, but there are general principles applicable to both and the remainder of this chapter, while referring to dementia generally, will be mainly concerned with Alzheimer's disease.

The Onset of Dementia

When a person becomes demented it will usually be noticed first by close friends and family. It would be rare for anyone to come to the conclusion quickly that a person was demented; more often what is noticed is a change of character or a loss of interest in something which was previously a feature of the person's life. It can also be the case that a previous skill will be lost. Examples from my own experience include the daily golfer who, for no apparent reason, gave up golf; the excellent cook who would miss vital ingredients out of recipes; the avid reader who no longer picks up a newspaper; the loving spouse who becomes aggressive and uncaring; and the inability to recognize friends and family, and a general loss of memory.

These are the early stages of the disease, and it depends upon the precise nature of the problems being experienced by the dementing person as to whether they or a relative seeks help from the medical services. Usually the general practitioner will be the first port of call. As the disease progresses there will be increasing reasons why the person may require, or through circumstances, come into contact with medical care. It may become obvious to relatives, as time passes, that something is seriously wrong with the person. The small changes in character and the episodes in which uncharacteristic mistakes are made may have initially been dismissed as 'old age' or 'forgetfulness'. However, as the disease progresses, all of these problems will become worse and additional features will become apparent, such as aimless wandering, 'turning night into day', severe loss of appetite or alternatively eating inappropriate, bizarre and disgusting items (such as pet food, pot plant soil and even faeces) instead of a proper diet (see Chapter 10). Aggression may lead to violence and it is quite possible that the patient will become incontinent. The course of events is unique for each person; it is not uncommon for someone suffering from dementia to be picked up by the police for wandering and endangering themselves or for shoplifting (caused by simply forgetting to pay), but it is usually the relatives who seek help.

It may be difficult to get the dementing person to accept that anything is wrong with them and even

harder to persuade them to attend a general practitioner's clinic, so it is quite common for a home visit,
for the purpose of assessing the patient, to be made.
The outcome of the eventual diagnosis of dementia,
which can be achieved by a combination of history
taking, observation, interview and administration of
mental tests (see Chapter 5), will depend on the
severity of the disease at the time of diagnosis, the
ability of the family to cope and the availability of
services—both social and nursing—in the person's
locality.

Family Support

The term 'dementia' conjures up many images in the
lay person and the fact of having a close relative
diagnosed as being demented is a devastating event
for any family. It is essential that those who are closest
to the dementing person, i.e. spouses and children,
and who may have a responsibility for continuing to
care for the person, are as fully informed as possible
about the likely outcome of the diagnosis. The nature
of dementia must be explained as clearly as possible
and backed up with readable and informative literature.
The fact that (at the time of writing) the disease is
irreversible must be emphasized, but it should also be
explained that this does not mean that many of the
aspects of the disease cannot be alleviated and that
routine medical complications cannot be dealt with.

It can help relatives to realize that the awful things
they are witnessing in their parent or spouse are not
unusual in dementia; this reinforces the feeling that
they are not alone. Towards this end, various groups
have been formed around the relatives and sufferers
of dementia, and it may be appropriate to give the

relatives the address of a nearby group or a national organization such as Scottish Action on Dementia (see Appendix). This should not be forced upon people, however, as some families are fiercely independent and some people do not want to share their experiences with others. For some relatives the time will come when they do want the support and opportunity to share with others who are going through the same experiences, and nurses, medical staff and social workers should establish such a relationship that they are able to offer such help when the time is right and the opportunity presents itself.

It should be borne in mind very much by professionals in contact with the relatives of dementia sufferers that the disease is progressive, that each day will bring new problems for the families and that established problems may well get worse. For this reason it is necessary to establish a relationship such that a watchful eye can be kept on the family and ongoing practical help offered at the right times.

The Effects on Family Life

The experience of a family with a member who has dementia has been described as 'premature bereavement' (Riggans, 1992). This is the case because, particularly in Alzheimer's disease, the person may ultimately undergo a complete change in character; old interests are completely forgotten; the closest of relatives, including spouses and children, are not recognized; the problems, particularly incontinence and wandering, may take such a heavy toll on the life of a family that normal life is impossible; and, finally, aggression and violence may be an ever-present threat. It is almost as if the old person is not there and someone new is present. This is a distressing concept, but it is also one that can help families to cope with the development of the disease; it may make it easier, ultimately, to seek further help, including long-term care, for their relative. The experiences of relatives who have lived with a demented person and tried to care for them need to be listened to closely by health-care and social-work professionals. The experience has been described by one writer as 'a living death' (Wood, 1990).

If a person comes into continuing care it is necessary to realize that, as hard as it is to care for them as professionals, we can go home at the end of our allotted span of duty. For relatives it has often been a 24-hour a day phenomenon and, for this reason, they have a lot to offer in the way of advice and information about the patient. It is necessary to listen to and implement sound advice from relatives; not only will this lead to a better standard of care for the patient but it will reassure relatives that the best level of care is being delivered, which will help them to feel that they still have a role to play in the life and care of the dementing person. Their feelings, which may include guilt at having their parent or spouse admitted to long-term care, should thus be alleviated.

The Demented Patient

The early stages of dementia, as they might be observed and described by someone close to a patient with dementia, have been discussed above. It is convenient to refer to this as stage 1 of dementia, and this is followed by stages 2 and 3. There is some overlap in the characteristics of the stages and the characteristics are not exclusive, but there are enough similarities between patients for this to be a reasonable classification. Stage 1 may last for from 2 to 4 years (Box 3.3).

Stage 2 is marked by a more rapid decline in the person's condition. Intellectual ability becomes markedly deteriorated with consequences such as inappropriate behaviour, wandering which may appear aimless to the onlooker but seems purposeful to the demented person, repetitive behaviour, which has been described as futile, further personality change and a complete inability, on behalf of the person, to carry out any activities of daily living without help. In other words, the person requires a high level of physical care. This stage of the disease may last for many years and, even if the condition is not deteriorating during this time, the sheer physical and mental strain begins to show on families and other carers

---

Stages of dementia

Stage 1
Memory loss, lack of spontaneity, subtle personality changes, disorientation to time and date

Stage 2
Impaired cognition and abstract thinking, restlessness and agitation, wandering, inability to carry out activities of daily living, impaired judgement, inappropriate social behaviour, lack of insight, repetitive behaviour, voracious appetite

Stage 3
Emaciation, indifference to food, inability to communicate, urinary and faecal incontinence, seizures

Box 3.3

who are trying to cope with the demented person at home.

Some of the problems have already been alluded to earlier in the chapter but it is worth considering them here in more detail. Taking continence as an example, it may be the case that a demented person, in stage 2 of the disease, is not strictly speaking incontinent of either urine or faeces. However, the decline in cognitive ability may be such that the person cannot remember how to find the toilet; even if the toilet is found or they are taken there by a carer, the person may not recognize the toilet for what it is. If the person is not taken to the toilet, he or she may mistake some other household object for the toilet. It is quite clear, if the above is the case, that the person cannot be left alone for significant periods of time. This contributes to a very real breakdown in family life as it may be impossible for family members, if they are alone with the person, to get out to the shops and to have any kind of social life. Inappropriate urination may become such a problem that the house begins to smell, so that the carers may be too embarrassed to have visitors, leading to further social isolation.

Wandering

One well-recognized problem in dementia during the second stage is wandering, although this term is somewhat vague; research into the types of wandering has been carried out (Hope & Fairburn, 1990). Wandering may simply involve ceaseless walking around the house. However, this can be disruptive for carers as it may continue both night and day. One danger for patients is that they are burning up enormous amounts of energy and, quite literally, exhausting themselves.

This may lead to sleeping at the wrong time for prolonged periods, for example in the middle of the day, and may contribute to the phenomenon of 'turning night into day'. Wandering poses further dangers for the person with dementia, however, and it may be the case that the demented person wanders away from home and becomes lost. If they are not properly clad on a cold day, one possible outcome of this could be hypothermia. The sense of the potential danger of traffic may be lost, with obvious consequences. One particular type of wandering which must be particularly difficult for carers to cope with is one whereby the demented person will constantly 'check up' on the carer to the extent that they may follow the carer around all the time, walking closely behind them.

Nutritional Aspects

Altered eating is also a well-recognized consequence of the cognitive decline associated with dementia (see Chapter 10; Morris et al, 1989). It has been postulated that this is a unique aspect of dementia since the kind of altered eating observed in dementia is not seen in other cognitive disorders. While a complete loss of appetite and the ability to feed is a feature of the terminal stages of dementia, in the second stage it can be the case that a person either loses their appetite or begins to overeat. The behaviour is usually totally inappropriate and may lead to either weight gain or weight loss. In the case of increased eating, the person may eat whole jars of jam or pickles or may begin to eat foods that they previously disliked. At its most disturbing, the behaviour may involve the eating of foods such as pet food, if it is left where the person can get a hold of it, and soil from pot plants or disgusting substances such as faeces. Obviously, this is extremely difficult for relatives who are caring for the demented person to cope with and may provide a further reason why the demented person cannot be left at home unattended.

Aggression

Aggression is not uncommon in stage 2 dementia and, again, it is associated with cognitive decline (Page, 1992). The demented person may misinterpret the actions of others, reflections in the mirror become 'intruders', and others may be accused of stealing things which the demented person has simply misplaced or never actually had. One general feature of the disease is that the person has a reduced ability to cope with stress and this can lead to complete mental breakdown on occasions due to the simplest matters, which would not have bothered the person before they became demented, becoming exaggerated.

Obviously, the transition into stage 3 dementia is not discrete; the problems apparent in stage 2 become progressively worse and, as time passes, more problems become manifest. Stage 3 is looked upon as being the terminal stage of dementia. It usually only lasts about 2 years but it can last much longer. The development of stage 3 is a common reason for admission of a demented person into long-term care, although this may have happened during stage 2. The decision to admit is not made on the basis of the person's decline into stage 3 alone. As mentioned above, the stages are not discrete enough to allow this. Inevitably, admission takes place because the burden for the carers at home has become too great or some specific crisis has occurred. It is not always the case that demented persons are admitted to long-term care; each case is unique.

The Terminal Stages

Stage 3 is characterized by almost total loss of cognitive ability, which leads to extreme apathy and an inability to communicate. The patient is quite likely to become incontinent of both urine and faeces and will completely lose interest in food and eating. It is often the case that the person will be totally dependent on the help of others for all activities of daily living, including feeding. There is a well-documented loss in body weight, even if an apparently adequate nutritional intake is being achieved, in demented patients. This is not fully understood but it should not necessarily be assumed that, because a demented person is losing weight that their nutritional intake is low relative to normal levels. This should also be explained to relatives who may think that the person is being deliberately underfed.

Nursing Care

Ideally, nursing care should begin as early as possible after the diagnosis of dementia has been made. This is not to imply that a high level of nursing care is required from the start or that all patients are going to come into care but rather it is aimed at establishing a relationship with the dementing person and the family in order that advice can be offered, future prospects explained, practical help given and, if possible, crisis averted. In the early stages it is very likely that a social worker will be involved and, indeed, some social-work facilities provide continuing care for highly dependent demented patients; nurses have no monopoly of care in this condition.

The aim of nursing care is to establish, at whatever stage of the disease the patient is first encountered, what abilities for activities of daily living remain and what residual cognitive ability remains. The initial aim is to maintain as much as possible of the patient's abilities, thereby maximizing independence and sustaining it for as long as possible. In this way, while the disease progresses, it is possible to slow down the decline in self-care ability, behaviour and cognitive ability. Decline in all abilities is inevitable, and nurses need to be aware of this in order to set realistic goals for individual patients, to know when it is really necessary to compensate, through nursing care, for a patient's lack of ability and to set new goals and implement new aspects of care. Some aspects of dementia have been investigated more than others and it is possible to report on the evaluation of the techniques of reality orientation and on the effect of exercise programmes.

Reality Orientation

Reality orientation is particularly important when an elderly person has been admitted to long-term care, not only to maintain a sense of time, space and identity but also, in many cases, to counteract the adverse effects of being in an institution. The subject of *institutionalization* will be dealt with in more depth in the chapter on *Continuing Care* (Chapter 7). It is all too easy for elderly patients in hospital or elderly residents in homes to be left for prolonged periods, starting very early in the morning, in a day room or sitting room in which the television is left permanently switched on. Often being unable to do anything about the television they may, as a result, be forced to listen to children's programmes or, in the evening, to 'Top of the Pops'. This would be very unlikely to be their choice of programme at home and inflicting such a diet on a confused elderly person can only hasten their decline from reality and increase their disorientation.

Reality orientation is an effort to maintain a sense of reality, in terms of time, space and person, in patients who are undergoing cognitive decline (Hanley et al, 1981). Reality orientation works at different levels—i.e. with individual patients or with groups—and can be implemented in various ways. Some of the measures used for reality orientation are quite common sense and involve labelling doors such as toilet doors and television room doors (Box 3.4). This does not necessarily have to be done with words; symbols can be used instead. Another strategy, aimed at groups of patients, is to have a notice-board and a clock in a position where it can easily be seen by all patients. Information such as the day and the date, along with any notable events or anniversaries, can be displayed on the board. Obviously, writing on the board has to

---

Features of reality orientation

Clocks set at correct time and visible
Orientation boards showing date, menu and daily events
Labels on doors, e.g. toilets, dining rooms, etc.
Group therapy
Constant orientation to environment

Box 3.4

be legible and a commitment has to be made to changing the information on the board daily in order for it to be of any value. Clocks have to be in good working order; if they stop for any reason it is probably better to remove them, and have them repaired or replaced quickly, than to leave a them permanently displaying the wrong time in the view of demented patients.

More sophisticated methods of reality orientation have been tested and there are two ways in which this can be done. Either patients are removed from their normal environment for classroom type sessions of reality orientation or they remain in their normal environment and are periodically oriented towards it. In the latter approach individual patients on a ward, for instance, can be taken by members of the nursing staff and walked round the ward, stopping at significant places such as the toilets and the dining rooms and being shown where they are. Both methods are effective in improving cognition but the latter approach is more effective in improving the behaviour of patients. It can be seen how this might be the case, because patients are being oriented to their environment in a way in which they can make sense of it and use it. They are also forming important bonds with members of the nursing staff.

Validation Therapy

Something which is often seen as being the opposite of reality orientation is validation therapy (Bleathman & Morton, 1988). This is not the case. Validation therapy is used under different circumstances and for different reasons from reality orientation, and the two can be used in the same environment and on the same patients. Validation therapy involves the exploration of a patient's feelings in order to attempt to steer him or her to reality or, at least, to an acceptance of the situation in which they find themselves. For example, if an elderly demented person tries to leave a safe, caring environment and claims to be looking for his or her mother, instead of immediately confronting them with the fact that their mother died years ago or (and this is considered to be very poor nursing practice) going along with the delusion, the nursing approach could be to ask the person about their mother; was she very close to the patient or when did the patient last see her?

Reminiscence Therapy

Along the lines of the above therapies, something which is used with older people generally and with demented patients particularly is reminiscence therapy. This is useful in stimulating the person to think about the past, to reveal more about their life to nursing staff or to therapists, and often just to enjoy a chat about how life used to be. As much as anything it may do for the patient, it often gives nursing staff a new insight into those for whom they are caring. None of the above therapies should be seen as being exclusive, nor should they be seen as being particularly time consuming or requiring expensive equipment or a high level of training. They should all be ongoing aspects of the care of demented patients which are practised by all nursing staff in care of the elderly.

Exercise Programmes

The loss of ability to perform self-care or activities of daily living is one aspect of dementia which has been investigated through the use of moderate exercise programmes (Jirovec, 1991). It has, in fact, been demonstrated that such programmes do increase the ability to self-care and they also reduce the incidence of urinary incontinence. In this light, the importance of walks round the hospital grounds and day trips and outings can be seen in the continuing treatment of demented patients; it is not always necessary to have a formal programme of exercises. This is very encouraging because it enables nursing staff to make sense of the care they are delivering. It will nearly always be the case that dramatic improvements do not take place. However, it can be shown that, without the care and activities in which nurses engage demented patients, that their condition would undoubtedly be worse. Nurses find caring for demented patients very stressful and it is important to be able to demonstrate that nursing care really makes a difference.

The environment in which the demented person is cared for has been shown to influence behaviour and also the course of cognitive decline (Berg et al, 1991). There is evidence to show that specialized units for demented patients offer an advantage in terms of slowing down cognitive decline. With reference to feeding, which is a problem in demented patients, it has been demonstrated that the decor of the room, the seating arrangements and the involvement of staff all influence the feeding of demented patients who are still able to feed themselves. The problem of assisted feeding in demented patients will be covered in more detail in the chapter on *Nutrition* (Chapter 10).

DEPRESSION

Depression is common in elderly people and, when the social circumstances, life events and physical problems of the elderly are examined it is possible to see why this may be so. The reason for including depression in this chapter is that depressed patients can often appear to be confused and, indeed, depression is often misinterpreted as dementia. The differential diagnosis can be difficult for a psychiatrist but generally speaking, and it is possible to test for this, mental faculties remain intact in the depressed patient, whereas the demented patient becomes increasingly cognitively impaired. Severely depressed patients, however, are often unresponsive and unable to feed, dress and maintain continence, and it can be seen how, without proper investigation, they can be considered to be demented. Signs of depression can include the following: agitation, restlessness and wandering at night, aimless wandering during the day, severe loss of appetite, constipation, loss of interest in self and surroundings, leading to neglect, confusion and failure to respond to other people, for example when asked a question.

There are two types of depression, either exogenous or reactive depression and endogenous depression. The former results from some identifiable cause such as an event in a person's life, for example bereavement, hospital admission, illness, or feelings of rejection by friends and relatives. In an elderly person this will probably have had a recent onset in later life. On the other hand, endogenous depression will probably have had an early onset in life. People with endogenous depression can be quite mentally disordered even experiencing delusions and often being suicidal.

Suicide is common in the elderly, especially among men, and all threats should be taken seriously.

With exogenous depression it is usually sufficient to support the patient though the period of depression such as after bereavement or during their stay in hospital. Sometimes it is possible to do something about the cause, for instance, ensuring that the elderly person who is afraid to return home after a stay in hospital, has sufficient support at home. It is rare for drug therapy, in the form of antidepressants, to be required. With endogenous depression, however, drug therapy is common and often effective but, in severe cases, treatment such as electroconvulsive therapy may be necessary (Branfield, 1992).

CONCLUSION

To conclude, therefore, the nursing care of demented patients offers one of the greatest challenges within the whole discipline of nursing. There is much that nursing staff can do to improve the life of a demented patient and the prospect of further research work into the problems of dementia offers great hope for the future.

REFERENCES

Berg L, Buckwalter KC, Chafetz PK, Gwyther LP, Holmes D, Koepke KM, Lawton MP, Lindeman DA, Magaziner J, Maslow K, Morley JE, Ory MG, Rabins PV, Sloane PD & Teresi J (1991) Special care units for persons with dementia. *Journal of the American Geriatrics Society* **39**:1229–1236.

Bleathman C & Morton I (1988) Validation therapy with the elderly. *Journal of Advanced Nursing* **13**:511–514.

Branfield M (1992) ECT for depression in elderly people. *Nursing Standard* **6**(26):24–26.

Eccles J & Wattis J (1988) Underlying physical causes of confusion in the elderly. *Geriatric Medicine* **18**(4):55–63.

Hanley IG, McGuire RJ & Boyd WD (1981) Reality orientation and dementia: a controlled trial of two approaches. *British Journal of Psychiatry* **138**(10):10–14.

Hope RA & Fairburn CG (1990) The nature of wandering in dementia: a community-based study. *International Journal of Geriatric Psychiatry* **5**:239–245.

Jirovec MM (1991) The impact of daily exercise on the mobility, balance and urine control of cognitively impaired nursing home residents. *International Journal of Nursing Studies* **28**(2):145–151.

Killeen J (1991) *Dementia in Scotland Agenda for Action*. Scottish Action on Dementia, Edinburgh.

Mackay A (1991) Subtypes of dementia. *Scottish Action on Dementia Annual Conference*, Glasgow, 24th June 1991.

Morris CH, Hope RA & Fairburn CG (1989) Eating habits in dementia. *British Journal of Psychiatry* **154**:801–806.

Page S (1992) Aggression in Alzheimer's disease. *Nursing Standard* **6**(24):37–39.

Riggans L (1992) Living with loss. *Nursing Times* **88**(27):34–35.

Thomas M (1990) Understanding the other dementias. *Scottish Action on Dementia Annual Conference*, Edinburgh, 22nd June 1990.

Wood C (1990) A living death. *Community Outlook*, June:30–31.

BIBLIOGRAPHY

Council on Scientific Affairs (1986) Dementia. *Journal of the American Medical Association* **256**(16):2234–2238.

A comprehensive look at the condition of dementia by an expert North American panel.

Crump A (1992) Restless spirits. *Nursing Times* **88**(21):26–28.

Wandering must be assessed in confused individuals before they can be helped.

Diesfeldt HFA & Diesfeldt-Groenendijk H (1977) Improving cognitive performance in psychogeriatric patients: the influence of physical exercise. *Age & Ageing* **6**:58–64.

A research article that shows that it is possible to measure improvements in demented subjects.

Dodwell D (1987) Alzheimer's disease: the clinical picture In Pitt B (ed.) *Dementia*. Churchill Livingstone, Edinburgh, pp. 174–176.

A chapter from a very good book on dementia which describes well the condition and its effect on the individual.

Emmerson C (1992) Fighting depression. *Nursing Times* **88**(17):60–62.

Describes the assessment of depression in elderly people and a 10-step process for helping elderly depressed patients.

Foreman MD (1989) Confusion in the hospitalised elderly: incidence, onset, and associated factors. *Research in Nursing & Health* **12**:21–29.

There are many reasons why the elderly become confused in hospital.

Nichols D (1991) *Mentally Disabled Adults*. Scottish Law Commission, Edinburgh.

A discussion document on advocacy for people who are mentally disabled, including those with dementia.

Richards BS (1990) Alzheimer's disease: a disabling neurophysiological disorder with complex nursing implications. *Archives of Psychiatric Nursing* **4**(1):39–42.

Written from the psychiatric nursing perspective.

Rogers RL, Meyer JS & Mortel KF (1990) After reaching retirement age physical activity sustains cerebral perfusion and cognition. *Journal of the American Geriatrics Society* **38**:123–128.

A research article which shows that it is possible to measure improvements in normal subjects.

Ryden MB, Bosenmaier M & McLachlan C (1991) Aggressive behaviour in cognitively impaired nursing home residents. *Research in Nursing & Health* **124**:87–95.

A survey of the problem and the situations in which it arises.

SECTION II: CARE OF THE ELDERLY SETTINGS

Chapter 4
Care in the Community

Most of the care of dependent older people in the community is carried out by families in the home of the older person. It is important to appreciate this and also to appreciate that community nursing services only reach a very small proportion of those elderly people in the community who require care, despite the fact that community nurses spend the majority of their time with older people.

Nursing care of the elderly in the community is mainly carried out by district nurses and involves a great many disciplines other than nursing; it also raises many issues which are quite different from those faced in the hospital setting. Collectively, the different professionals involved in delivering care in the community are known as the Primary Health Care Team. The core of the team is comprised of the general practitioner, the health visitor, the district nurse, supported by nursing auxiliaries, and also specialists such as continence advisers and stoma care nurses. Also involved in community care of older people are the community psychiatric nurse and members of the Community Mental Health Team.

There are, therefore, good reasons for looking at this area of care of the elderly, because of these different clinical issues and also because of government legislation which is attempting to encourage greater use of the community in the care of elderly people. Proposed changes in nurse training are leading to an emphasis on this particular area of care and its further development as a speciality within nursing.

Community nursing presents some problems for the nurse. For a start, it is a completely different environment from the hospital and one in which nurses may feel less in control of the situations which are encountered. On the whole, patient care is carried out in the individual patient's home and, apart from issues of who is in control, the environment may be wholly unsuitable or may need adapting in order for certain procedures (e.g. asceptic technique) to be carried out.

GOVERNMENT POLICY

The increasing number of elderly people and the concomitant rise in those who require medical and nursing care means that the resources of the health service are becoming more stretched. In particular, this pressure is felt in hospitals, where there never appear to be sufficient numbers of beds for the assessment, rehabilitation and continuing care of older people. One way of relieving this pressure and obviating the need for more hospital building is to shift the burden of care, to an even greater extent, from the hospital into the community and to concentrate resources there. One of the objectives in achieving this is to keep people out of hospital for as long as possible and to hospitalize only when it is absolutely necessary. In the meantime, people will be cared for at home with adequate nursing and social services backing and support for the relatives and families who will provide the bulk of the care in the home. This thinking was encapsulated in the United Kingdom in the *Griffiths Report* of 1988 (Griffiths, 1988).

Being cared for at home has many advantages for the individual elderly person. The surroundings and the faces are familiar and the fear of becoming institutionalized is lessened. However, the possibility of institutionalization (to be discussed in the chapter on *Continuing Care*; Chapter 7) is still present. The nurse working with elderly people in the community should be aware of this and try to lessen its impact by ensuring that an 'institution' is not set up within the older person's own home and run for the benefit of the family and the care staff who visit.

THE WORK OF THE DISTRICT NURSE

It is necessary for nurses in hospital, who are working with older people, to be reminded occasionally that the majority (95%) are living in the community and have no requirement for hospital care. Many of those in the community are well, but the increasing number of older people *per se* and the increase in physical and mental disorders with age means that a great deal of nursing is carried out in the community.

It has already been established that older people tend to have more than one medical condition and, therefore, require more medical care. This is reflected in a greater number of visits to the general practitioner by the older person and by a greater level of drug prescribing to older people generally. It is not surprising to find, therefore, that the work of the district nurse is taken up largely by elderly people. It has been estimated that 75% of the time of the district nurse is spent with older people.

The work of the district nurse has been outlined as shown in Box 4.1. It can be seen that, for all of the points outlined in Box 4.1, older people can provide the majority of clients.

Assessment

The work of the district nurse begins, not unnaturally, with the assessment of clients, and Box 4.2 gives an outline of the principles upon which this assessment

---

The work of the district nurse

1 Identification of physical, emotional and social needs of patients in their own homes, as well as the wider needs of the community

2 Planning and provision of appropriate programmes of nursing care particularly for the following groups; the chronically sick, disabled, frail elderly, terminally ill and post-operative patients

3 Mobilizing community resources, both professional and voluntary

4 Identification of the special needs of the carer and family

5 Ensuring continuity of care between home and hospital in both directions

6 Promotion of health education and self-care with individuals and groups

7 Rehabilitation

8 Counselling

Box 4.1

Principles of assessment of elderly people in the community

A continuous cycle of assessment and reassessment

Assessment of the carer's needs alongside the patient's

Assessment starting from the patient or carer's concerns

Access to information from other agencies/professionals

Multidisciplinary assessment

Acknowledgement of intuitive and subjective assessment

Box 4.2

should be based (Ross, 1991). As described in the introduction to this chapter, the nurse in the community is in quite a different position from the nurse in hospital. Whether or not one subscribes to patient-centred care, it is always the case that the nurse in the hospital is in a more powerful position *vis-à-vis* patients than in the community. The district nurse is 'a guest in the patient's home, with no right of entry. The patient therefore has ultimate authority and can play a major role in negotiation for change' (Ross, 1991). Information is gathered in very different, and perhaps more imaginative and less formal ways, than the way in which it is done in hospital. This is illustrated by the following quote from Ross (1991).

Important information is obtained on the doorstep at

the first visit. The appearance, access to the property and state of the garden give useful clues. The response when the doorbell rings—whether there is the noise of boisterous children, a dog barking or a long silence followed by the shuffle of bedroom slippers—should also be noted. This, combined with the person's expression of anxiety, relief, fatigue or despair contribute to the nurse's assessment.

The assessment has to be translated into a plan for care, and this must be done with the full cooperation of the patient. It is not unusual for a record of the patient's care to be kept in the home, as well as another record at the centre where the district nurse works. This has implications for the way in which records are kept and what is stated in them. It has to be borne in mind that the patient or a relative can read the nursing notes and recordings; this is very different from the situation which generally prevails in hospital.

In assessing an elderly person at home there are indexes available whereby the district nurse can ask about normal daily activities and rate the patient for ability to maintain independence. Such a scale is the Shanas Functional Capacity Index (Box 4.3). This index can be completed by questioning the individual or by proxy information obtained from a spouse or other relative (Henderson & McConnel, 1990).

Planning Care

Planning care and taking action as a district nurse often involves a high level of decision making and, since district nurses work alone, they have fewer contacts or colleagues with whom to share problems and help with decision making. One major problem

---

Shanas Functional Capacity Index

Can the patient:
1 Go out of doors
2 Walk up and down stairs
3 Get about the house
4 Wash and bathe self
5 Dress self and put on shoes
6 Cut own toenails?

Does the patient do this:
Without difficulty and without assistance?
With some difficulty, but without assistance of
another person?
With difficulty and only with assistance of another
person?

Box 4.3

appears to be the decision on when to stop visiting
an elderly patient who no longer requires any nursing
care. The visits in the past may have engendered a
sense of dependency upon the district nurse and, when
the aim of the district nurse is to promote the
independence of the patient, their actions may seem
to conflict with this and lead to problems. The district
nurse needs to have a good knowledge of the family
situation of the elderly person in their care and thereby
know what faces them when care is withdrawn; do
they face loneliness and a decline in their physical and
mental state or will the family rally round? The part
which the social-work department can play and the
role of local voluntary organizations needs to be
understood and, in many cases, the district nurse may

be the one to advise an elderly person or to make contact with other organizations.

THE COMMUNITY/HOSPITAL INTERFACE

It may appear, at times, that the only choice to be made is between care in a hospital or care at home, in the community. This is not the case; there are several ways in which care in the home can be backed up by hospital and hospital-type services which are, fundamentally, aimed at keeping people at home for as long as is reasonably possible. In this chapter we will look at two systems for such care—the day hospital and respite care.

Older people have been shown to be particularly vulnerable at what has been described as the community/hospital interface (Young et al, 1991). The reasons for this result from lack of policy about admission to and discharge from hospital, and the outcome of this is that there is poor planning and poor communication. Ultimately, elderly people in the community become more dependent without this being picked up by general practitioners and, therefore, community nurses. One way in which this is overcome by some health authorities is the creation of the post of geriatric liaison health visitor, a health visitor who has the job of specifically visiting older people in the community and helping to plan admissions and also discharges in such a way that the support services can be used effectively on behalf of the dependent elderly person.

Further recommendations have been made in one report, which aim to improve the movement of dependent older people between home and hospital.

Such recommendations include an agreed admission and discharge policy; multidisciplinary training of staff on local resources for elderly people; communication with the Primary Health Care Team (general practitioner services) when someone is admitted to hospital or dies in hospital; minimizing unnecessary transfer of elderly patients within hospital once they are admitted; having specialized teams to work with older people and the creation (for the future) of a generic community worker.

THE DAY HOSPITAL

The day hospital will often be part of a larger local hospital and will usually be staffed by nurses who work only daytime hours during the week. The day hospital functions in such a way that elderly people who require quite a high degree of care can visit usually once a week, though visits can be more or less frequent as the situation demands. Patients can be given some nursing care which is difficult or impossible to give at home, such as a bath or shower or nail trimming, and they can also be assessed for any deterioration in general condition. In this way it is possible on a weekly basis, depending on the size of the day hospital, to deliver care and come into contact with many more patients than if they were admitted for longer stays.

The time spent at the day hospital is also an ideal opportunity for treatment and assessment by physiotherapists and occupational therapists. It is also a good opportunity for the geriatrician to see the patient.

RESPITE CARE

Respite care can be viewed as being for the beneift of informal carers (friends and relatives) as much as for the benefit of the elderly person who is receiving it. However it is viewed, the objective is again to help to keep the elderly person who requires care at home for as long as possible. Respite care involves periodic admission for a week or a fortnight at regular intervals— dictated by individual need—into a care of the elderly unit. In this way, informal carers can have an opportunity for rest and even to get away on holiday. The latter should definitely be encouraged by nursing staff as daily visits to the hospital by the relatives will defeat the purpose of respite care.

The transition from home to hospital can be difficult, even for the short lengths of stay associated with respite, and some preparation and support is required for both the person being admitted and also for the relatives. Feelings of guilt can arise in relatives who are leaving an elderly person in hospital. It may be the case that the respite patient is also a day-hospital patient, so some liaison can be established between staff in the two locations and pre-admission visits can be arranged. It is often rumoured that patients are more likely to die when they come into respite care, but research work indicates that this is not true (Pearson, 1988).

While a patient is in respite care it is possible to carry out some assessment procedures from the nursing and medical point of view. A full medical examination can be carried out and some aspects of nursing care can be assessed. Problems such as pressure sores and difficulty in managing incontinence can be tackled, though these have to be approached in a realistic way since the patient will be returning home where the kind of equipment that is used in hospital may not be available. If the carers are obviously struggling to care for the elderly person then some liaison with the district nurse may be possible, either to obtain another angle on the situation, if the district nurse is already involved in the case, or to call in the district nurse in cases where the need for more support is indicated.

From the nursing point of view, respite care has many advantages. In a continuing care environment, where most of the patients are unlikely to be discharged, it provides another angle on care of the elderly. In cases where the person has eventually to be admitted for continuing care, a rapport between the staff and the patient and relatives will already have been established and, in this way, admission for continuing care is less traumatic.

THE FUTURE OF COMMUNITY CARE

As there has been an increasing emphasis in recent years on community care, through government legislation and, by the professional services, of which nursing is only one example, it is worth considering what the future holds and looking at the available research and the issues which it raises. So far, we have only considered the role of the nurse in the community but we will now widen the discussion to include the informal carers, and their requirements, and the role of other services, principally the social services.

Obviously, as the focus of care of the elderly moves from the hospital to the community this will put an increasing burden upon the informal carers. Informal carers include the spouses, immediate family, and sometimes friends and neighbours of the dependent elderly person. There is often great resistance on the part of an elderly person to being admitted to hospital; this is hardly surprising since it must seem preferable to be cared for in familiar surroundings and by familiar faces. Similarly, there is often equally tough resistance on the part of the informal carers to have a dependent elderly person admitted to hospital. Admission is often accompanied by a sense of guilt and a feeling that the elderly person has been 'let down', especially if he or she did not want to be admitted.

The Effects of Demographic Changes

The decreasing availability of hospital services for the elderly, relative to their increasing proportion in the population, means that there is an increasing burden of care being carried by the informal carers in the community. However willingly this care is undertaken it is essential that the informal carers receive the right social support and also adequate training for the kind of care they are being called upon to deliver at home. Very dependent elderly people are often cared for in very inadequate conditions and it has been shown that there are deficiencies in the kind of training which the informal carers are receiving. Research has demonstrated, for example, that informal carers receive adequate training in communicating with elderly people and dealing with confusion but rarely get adequate training in the more physical aspects of care, such as lifting and personal hygiene. Supporting informal carers in the community, therefore, requires that programmes of training and support specifically address their needs (Atkinson, 1992).

INTEGRATION OF HEALTH AND SOCIAL CARE

The community nurse liaises with others from the nursing, medical and paramedical professions but also with social care agencies organized by the local authority and with voluntary organizations. The community nurse requires, at least, a working knowledge of what these different agencies do and, whenever necessary, how they can be called upon for help.

Social Services

The home-help service provides help for elderly people at home with domestic tasks around the home such as cleaning, shopping and even preparation of meals. It will sometimes be the case that the visit of the community nurse will coincide with that of the home help and a relationship can be established. The home help is a key person in alerting the social services of the requirement for further support and also for alerting the general practitioner, thereby initially calling in the district nurse.

Meals

Another vital service to many elderly people at home is that of 'meals-on-wheels'; the responsibility for preparing and delivering this is shared between local authorities and voluntary organizations. This service ensures that certain dependent older people receive at least one hot meal that is nutritionally adequate at least once every few days and, in some cases, daily. An alternative to this home delivery service, and sometimes integrated with it, is the social day centre. This is not designed, as is the day hospital, to deliver nursing care but as a place where older people can go for a cooked lunch and also a bath, if necessary, and where other services such as chiropody can be supplied.

Benefits

Several benefits are available to elderly people on low incomes and, while it is the responsibility of the social services to advise on benefits, it may be possible for the community nurse to see a need and to direct the older person or their informal carers towards any of those shown in Box 4.4. Mainly, however, the district nurse should be directing people to their local social security offices or Citizens' Advice Bureau (Rundle & Broughton, 1991).

Voluntary Organizations

Voluntary organizations, and these include The Red Cross, Age Concern and the Women's Royal Voluntary Service (WRVS), can provide help with quite a variety of things depending on how they are organized locally. Of a more specialized nature are groups set up to support individuals and carers looking after certain

---

Social security benefits for the elderly

Attendance allowance

Invalid care allowance

Income support

Housing benefit

Box 4.4

conditions such as Parkinson's disease, Alzheimer's disease and stroke. In some cases, such bodies are organized on a national basis and, in other cases, they are only locally organized.

The best care, from both the health and social perspectives, is obviously delivered when the local authority and the local health authority work together. Some projects in which nursing staff and social-work staff work in the same setting, each giving their own particular care as required, are already underway. The collaboration between health and local authorities in the training of home-care aides is also taking place.

Making Referrals

It is essential, nevertheless, that all workers in the social- and health-care milieu within the community know how and when to make appropriate referrals. This is not dependent upon expertise in both disciplines, rather on the recognition of risk factors that indicate the need for either health or social care. Box 4.5 gives an example of some indicators for health care which could be used by a social-care worker or by a generic support worker to direct the appropriate services towards the dependent elderly person. By this means, a diagnosis is not arrived at, merely an indication of actual deterioration and potential risk.

Similarly, a scheme has been proposed whereby the need for social care might be indicated; it includes questions about the elderly person and the principal carer. The scheme looks, initially, at whether the person lives alone and how they are managing, and then looks at the principal carer and asks how available they are and how well they are coping (Silvey, 1991). Further assessment, either social or medical, requires special-

---

Indicators for health referral

Observed	**Told or heard**
Bruises—skin lesions	Pain
Pressure sores	Tiredness
Self neglect	Weight loss
Many pills	Falls or faints
	Speech difficulty
	Recent personality change
	Confusion: conversation/ behaviour
	Loss of appetite
	Loss of interest
	Changes in sleep pattern
	Loss of sexual drive

Observed/told or heard
Continence problems
Loss of physical independence in daily living
Poor muscular coordination or any limb weakness
Sensory failings
Alcohol excess
Sadness/tearfulness

Box 4.5

ized practitioners; and this is largely covered in the chapter on *Assessment* (Chapter 5).

CONCLUSION

It is very hard to do justice to the work of those who care for older people in the community, in terms of both its scope and importance, in a chapter of this length. The work of the district nurse has been outlined and some of the interface settings have also been described. Increasing deterioration in the condition of an elderly person in the community or an acute episode of disease can necessitate further assessment in order to determine whether a higher level of support is required in the community or in hospital. This forms the subject material of the following chapter.

REFERENCES

Atkinson FI (1992) Experience of informal carers providing nursing support for disabled dependants. *Journal of Advanced Nursing* **17**:835–840.

Griffiths R (1988) *Community Care: Agenda for Action. A Report to the Secretary of State for Social Services.* HMSO, London.

Henderson ML & McConnel ES (1990) Gerontological care in community settings. In Matteson MA & McConnel ES (eds) *Gerontological Nursing Concepts and Practice.* WB Saunders, Philadelphia, pp. 763–792.

Pearson ND (1988) An assessment of relief hospital admissions for elderly patients with dementia. *Health Trends* **20**:120–121.

Ross FM (1991) Nursing old people in the community. In Redfern S (ed.) *Nursing Elderly People.* Churchill Livingstone, Edinburgh, pp. 465–484.

Rundle R & Broughton H (1992) Social security benefits *Nursing Standard* **6**(39)(suppl):3–8.

Silvey J (1991) *Co-operation in Community Care.* University of Nottingham School of Social Studies, Nottingham.

Young E Wallace P & Victor C (1991) *Older People at the Interface.* St Mary's Hospital, Helen Hamlyn Research Unit, London.

BIBLIOGRAPHY

Department of Health Nursing Division (1989) *A Strategy for Nursing.* Department of Health, London.

This is worth reading in relation to any area of nursing and also contains paragraphs which are very pertinent to nursing in the community.

Henwood M (1992) *Through a Glass Darkly: Community Care and Elderly People.* Kings Fund, London.

This is a thoroughly comprehensive review of all the issues surrounding care of elderly people in the community.

Ross FM (1991) Nursing old people in the community. In Redfern S (ed.) *Nursing Elderly People.* Churchill Livingstone, Edinburgh, pp. 465–484.

An excellent chapter, already referred to in the text, which looks at community care from the perspective of the district nurse, but which also continues to look at other issues including social care.

Shaw MW (1984) Domiciliary care. In Shaw MW (ed.) *The Challenge of Ageing.* Churchill Livingstone, Melbourne, pp. 114–125.

Written from an Australian perspective, but many issues are relevant to the UK. Good on the occupational therapy side of community care.

United Kingdom Central Council for Nursing, Midwifery and Health Visiting (1991) *Report on Proposals for the Future of Community Education and Practice.* UKCC, London.

A detailed look at the areas within the community in which nurses work and the issues which this raises, particularly the need for more specific education of nurses for working in the community.

Chapter 5
Assessment

The concept of assessment, while not unique to care of the elderly, is very important in this discipline because the problems faced by older people who are ill are not just the sum of their physical problems or their medical diagnoses. For the elderly person who is ill there will be an accompanying range of psychological and social circumstances which will have a bearing on the outcome of their contact with the medical and nursing services. Because the care of an elderly person may represent a situation that has been ongoing for a number of years, assessment serves different functions. It can lead to an immediate plan for treatment and care of an elderly person and it can also serve to indicate how and where they should be most appropriately cared for: either long-term care (continuing care in hospital, nursing home or rehabilitation) or in the community with appropriate support.

Assessment is not the preserve of any one medical or paramedical discipline; rather, it is an area where several disciplines work together in order to establish as comprehensive a picture as possible of the individual elderly person. Assessment can take place in any environment. For reasons that will be discussed below, the normal home of the elderly person is the most ideal environment for assessment, but there are specifically designated 'assessment wards' within the geriatric medical services of health authorities. While these wards rarely deal solely with assessment they should, ideally, be the wards onto which the older people with problems requiring admission to hospital are admitted. it is on these wards that there is a concentration of the disciplines which can contribute towards assessment. Assessment, by its very nature, should be a continuous process and it should take place on all wards for care of the elderly. It is important, nevertheless, that an emphasis is placed upon assessment in the early stages of admission so that the elderly person requiring long-term care is appropriately placed.

Needs and Abilities

The process of assessment is not an entirely negative one. It may seem that all of the assessment environments and tools which are presented here are concerned with identifying problems which the older person may have. To some extent this is true but it is also the case that the residual abilities of the elderly person should be identified; in other words, what can the person still do independently and how little, regarding some aspects of care, does the nurse really have to do? Residual ability should not only be concerned with the physical aspects of daily living but also with the psychological. Does the elderly person have the will to carry out their own care and to try and improve their ability to care for themselves? The nurse is ideally placed, within the multidisciplinary team, to identify these abilities in the individual and thereby to help the team to arrive at a proper assessment of needs for the purposes of rehabilitation (the subject of the next chapter).

THE ASSESSMENT WARD

Assessment wards are ideally situated within a general hospital. There are several reasons for this. It may be the case that an elderly person has entered hospital routinely or through the emergency services. In either of these cases, they will not immediately come under the care of a geriatrician, even if they have previously required the services of the geriatric team.

During their admission to a general medical or surgical ward, or to any other specialized ward, it may become apparent that the elderly person is going to find it difficult coping at home. This may be directly as a result of their condition or because the family have intimated that they can no longer envisage coping with the person at home. It is convenient, in this case, that the geriatric assessment ward is co-located within the general hospital because, in order to facilitate the assessment, the elderly person can then be transferred within the hospital. This is less traumatic than being moved to another hospital but it is not always possible. Even if the elderly person has to be moved to another hospital for assessment then there are good reasons for having the assessment ward within a general hospital. The general hospital should be where the majority of the services required for a comprehensive assessment are located, and these include all of the services such as radiography, electrocardiography and audiology as well as physiotherapy and even social work and occupational therapy.

In some cases an older person will require psychiatric assessment. This may take place as part of a routine physical and social assessment or it may be necessary to admit the elderly person to a specialized unit, which will usually be located within a psychiatric hospital.

The details of psychiatric assessment are considered to be beyond the scope of this text; however, one of the screening tools for cognitive impairment, which may indicate that psychiatric assessment is required, is given later in this chapter.

The Assessment Nurse

The assessment ward should have a more 'homely' atmosphere than a general ward, as patients may have to spend considerable lengths of time there. Once assessment is complete, and if it indicates that continuing care is required, it may be several weeks before a suitable place becomes available. The nursing staff should be motivated towards the concept of assessment and should see their work as very much part of a process that will result in the patients in their care passing through and finding appropriate placements outwith the assessment ward. They should see the importance of their work; as in other care of the elderly environments, the nursing staff will be the key point of liaison between several disciplines. Nurses in this position can ensure that the assessment period goes as smoothly as possible for the patient by attending to the timetable of the assessment. This can practically be achieved by seeing that patients do not have to rush between appointments and that, if they simply do not feel up to attending a session with a particular therapist, they do not have to. In this case, the nurse should find out why and make arrangements for another session.

The older person undergoing assessment will be anxious. This anxiety will not only be about their physical condition but about what the future is going to hold. Nursing staff should ensure that elderly people are kept as informed as their mental state will allow and, if the person is unable to fully comprehend what is going on, then the relatives and significant friends should be kept as informed as possible. This is particularly important where a recommendation for ongoing care in some other environment is made, be it in continuing care or in a nursing home, as the elderly person and the family will want to come to some agreement as to the most suitable place. While the consultant will be ultimately responsible for making the placement or recommendation, it may be possible for nursing staff to arrange for visits to local nursing homes and even to continuing-care wards. For these reasons, the nursing staff need to be informed about the local facilities for long-term care, in order to help the older people and their families with any questions which they may have. This is not an area for expressed prejudices about private sector versus National Health Service or local authority homes, rather it is an area for nurses to be aware of what is best for the individual, what is affordable for the families concerned and for accurate information on the particular suitability of particular establishments for particular individuals.

Equipment

A final note about the assessment ward is that it should be no less well equipped than any other area for care of the elderly. The assessment ward is liable to admit patients who are very physically dependent and equipment will be required for their ambulation and other activities of daily living. If the ward is not well equipped—and I am referring to such basic equipment as ambulifts, lifting slings and adapted cutlery—then it will be quite possible to find out what the patient is not capable of doing but not possible to find out precisely how to overcome this difficulty. It is also of immense help, particularly in continuing care, if a patient who is admitted with particular deficits also comes with some suggestions on how the nursing staff can tackle these.

It is the responsibility of the nursing staff in assessment wards to ensure that there is a wide range of equipment which is well maintained and which other nursing staff are capable of using. Assessment wards are often not dedicated to this particular function; it is often convenient to combine the functions of assessment and rehabilitation, for obvious reasons; however, rehabilitation will be dealt with in Chapter 6.

THE ASSESSMENT AND PLANNING TEAM

It is not possible to give a definitive description of an assessment team as this would run counter to the whole concept and, indeed, the philosophy of assessment. It is possible, however, to indicate the usual, or perhaps the minimum, members of the team. It is necessary to emphasize that these core members should always be ready and willing to involve whichever other discipline is necessary in order to establish as comprehensive a picture of the individual elderly person as possible.

It is important, however, that the multidisciplinary team share the same philosophy and a useful starting point would be to see their common purpose as being concerned with the individual person rather than with a process through which some elderly people pass. Such a philosophy could be drawn up on a common basis and published for members of the multidisciplinary team to refer to in their work. The concept of statements of philosophy is dealt with in more detail in the chapter on *Continuing Care* (Chapter 7). Having such a shared purpose is not necessarily prescriptive of any particular model of care. Rather, it is concerned with putting the individual elderly person at the centre of the assessment process and ensuring that the aims of the process and the resulting goals for rehabilitation are drawn up with the consent and involvement of the elderly person, as far as is reasonably possible.

The 'Key Worker' Concept

A useful point at which to begin is the identification of one member of the assessment team as the 'key worker'. There is always some difficulty in doing this, as the 'key worker' requires definition and there are always interprofessional considerations to be taken into account. It should be emphasized that the key worker is not necessarily the leader of the assessment team; rather, he or she is the person who is most likely to initiate the assessment process and who is going to be kept best informed about the progress of the assessment. In most cases, therefore, the key worker can be considered to be the elderly person's general practitioner. The team is also referred to here as the assessment *and* planning team, as it is assumed that in arriving at a conclusion about the elderly person's abilities and circumstances that some recommendations will be made about future accommodation and care. Which team member is the key worker, therefore, may well change as the elderly person progresses through a process of assessment and placement in some alternative care environment; it is worth emphasizing that the real 'leader' of the assessment team is the individual elderly person, and it is their needs which will dictate the course of the assessment and planning procedures.

The General Practitioner

The general practitioner, having access to a detailed medical history, is ideally placed to be the key worker for an elderly person in the community. The elderly person may have been a patient for many years and, even if this is not the case, the medical notes which are held by the general practitioner will cover the whole medical history of the individual. Furthermore, the general practitioner is liable to know of the individual living circumstances of the elderly person either through first hand knowledge gained from home visits or through the district nurses working in the practice. On this basis the general practitioner will be able to recommend continued visits by the district nurse or an assessment by the social-work department, possibly by a medical social worker. Assessment by a social worker can reveal whether there are any needs for which benefits can be obtained, in order to help the older person at home, or whether further action is required.

The district nurse is an invaluable source of information about older people, even if visits are not currently being made. The district nurse will know if the elderly person will have difficulty in their present home and whether or not the spouse or family are able to cope with the elderly person as their condition deteriorates. Another worker, in the community whose services the general practitioner can call upon is the health visitor or, if there is one in the community, the geriatric liaison health visitor, who can carry out a detailed assessment of the health problems, if any, of the elderly person and the risks attendant in their home circumstances.

The Geriatrician

If an age-related illness is the problem from which the elderly person is suffering then the general practitioner can call on more specialized colleagues to make an assessment and to give their recommendations. For instance, a geriatrician could be asked to make a domiciliary visit in order to visit the person in their own home. If there is some obvious mental disability, then either the general practitioner or the geriatrician can make a referral to a psychiatrist. Again, in the case of an elderly person, it may be possible to make this a domiciliary visit.

It has already been mentioned that the most suitable place in which to make an assessment of an elderly person is at home. This is the case because it is in the home that the true abilities and limitations of the individual can be seen. The future for the ill elderly person depends not only on individual ability and problems but also on the environment in which they normally live. A key aspect of this environment may be the ability of the spouse or other significant family members and friends to cope with the elderly person on their own. To illustrate this, a moderately disabled elderly person may be able to continue to live at home if that home is suitable and if their spouse can cope with them and help them with some routine care tasks. On the other hand, if the home is unsuitable, then a change of environment may be indicated.

Having said, however, that assessment is best made in the patient's home, this may not always be possible to carry out. This may be the case for a number of reasons, and in this light it is worth mentioning that all of this section on the assessment and planning team could equally well be applied in hospital, in an assessment ward, with visits home for, for example, occupational-therapy assessment as and when required.

The Therapists

A very important element of the assessment and planning is carried out by the 'therapists' who can be asked to make an assessment by the general practitioner or who may be asked to do so by the geriatrician. This group of specialists includes the physiotherapists, occupational therapists and speech therapists. The dietitian may also be included at this stage. The purpose of the physiotherapist, as regards assessment of older people, is to assess physical function with respect to posture, walking, transferring and use of the upper limbs. The physiotherapist, of course, will also be able to make recommendations about whether or not the elderly person is liable to benefit from a course of physiotherapy designed to improve physical function. This assessment is, therefore, of great importance.

The Occupational Therapist The occupational therapist has the job of assessing how the individual elderly person's physical limitations influence their ability to carry out the activities of daily living, such as eating, toileting, washing and dressing. The occupational therapist can then suggest aids such as adapted feeding utensils, strategically placed hand rails and other design features of, for example, the kitchen, which will enable the elderly person to remain independent in their own environment. It may also be the case that the occupational therapist will come to the conclusion that the elderly person is unable to carry out activities of daily living in such a way that they can live independently. It is unusual for the speech therapist to be involved at this stage of the assessment, but they may be required to assess oral functioning and swallowing and to institute a course of training to help improve these functions. The community dietitian may be able to assess whether there is a nutritional deficiency, determining how this may have arisen and suggesting a course of action, such as dietary modification or supplements, in order to correct it. The work of the dietitian and the related nutritional responsibilities of the nurse will be covered in the chapter on *Nutrition* (Chapter 10).

FUNCTIONAL ASSESSMENT TOOLS

Precisely what normal ageing is, in terms of health and function, has never been adequately defined. In the absence of specific criteria, the assessment team can establish if there have been any deviations and deterioration from what the individual elderly person or relatives consider to be normal for that person. This, however, is only one aspect of assessment.

The assessment team normally tries to look at a range of functions including physical health, activities of daily living, psychological status and social status. By applying objective criteria to these various functions the assessment team can arrive at a composite picture of how the individual is managing in the face of ageing and disease and, using these criteria, can plan for the future.

A number of tools have been validated for the measurement of functional status in older people and a few of these will be considered here. As a general principle, regarding assessment tools, it is necessary to say that very few, if any, of these are perfect. For this reason, it is advisable to have expert guidance in interpreting the measurements made by these scales, and not to base an assessment and plan of care on only one tool. On the whole, the assessment tools try to provide the assessment team with a numerical score, or index, whereby the individual can be placed on a scale of, for example, ability/disability or mental function/incapacity. In order, therefore, to use such tools and to interpret them correctly, it is necessary for the the person, or the team, using them to understand fully what is being asked and to know how the particular index is derived from the tool and applied to the planning of care. Naturally, the tools are not unique to assessment, and they can also be used in rehabilitation in order to measure the progress of an individual who is undergoing a course of treatment or therapy. We will look, in turn, at five tools which measure physical condition, activities of daily living, instrumental activities of daily living, mental capacity and social status. Other tools will be considered in the chapter on *Rehabilitation* (Chapter 6).

PULSES Profile

The PULSES profile (Granger et al, 1979; Box 5.1) is a scale which measures physical condition and function by looking generally at physical condition and at the function of different systems as well as the requirement for physical support. Each of these functions is rated

---

Factors assessed by the PULSES profile

Physical condition
Includes diseases of the viscera (cardiovascular, gastrointestinal, urological and endocrine) and neurological disorders

Upper limb functions
Self-care activities (drink/feed, dress upper/lower, brace/prosthesis, groom, wash, perineal care), dependent mainly on upper limb function

Lower limb function
Mobility (transfer chair/toilet/tub or shower, walk, stairs, wheelchair), dependent mainly on lower limb function

Sensory components
Relating to communication (speech and hearing) and vision

Excretory functions
Bladder and bowel

Support factors
Consider intellectual and emotional adaptability, support from family unit and financial ability

---

Box 5.1

from 1 to 4 and a composite score, based on the sum of the scores for individual components in the scale, is obtained. It should be noted, in the use of this scale, that a low score indicates good condition and a high score indicates poor condition.

The Katz Index of Activities of Daily Living (ADL)

The Katz Index of ADL (Box 5.2) looks at six activities of daily living—bathing, dressing, toileting, transfer, continence and feeding—and assesses the ability of the individual to perform these independently. The individual is then placed on a position on the index such as 'requires assistance with transfer', and this position gives a definitive description of the individual whereby they can be described as being, for example, able to feed and maintain continence but have difficulty in transferring (Katz & Akpom, 1976). The individual will be independent or only partly require assistance in bathing and dressing. It is possible to place the individual in this way because the research on which the Katz Index of ADL is based established the sequence in which the ability to perform activities of daily living are lost with disability. Conversely, this research also established how independence in the activities of daily living is regained in the rehabilitative process.

Factors assessed in the Katz Index of Activities of Daily Living (ADL)

Bathing

Dressing

Going to the toilet

Transfer

Continence

Feeding

Box 5.2

Further to Katz's ADL are the Instrumental Activities of Daily Living (IADL) and these can be measured by the Scale for the IADL (Lawton & Brody, 1969; Box 5.3). The Scale for the IADL measures how disability or illness influences the ability of the individual to carry out practical tasks such as using the telephone and preparing food. An interesting refinement of the scale is that it gives different weightings to certain tasks for males and females, based on which tasks they are liable to be more accustomed to carry out. It will be interesting to see if these weightings need to be changed in the future as the traditional male role changes. The interpretation of this score is left to the occupational therapist administering it.

Factors assessed for Instrumental Activities of Daily Living (IADL)

Ability to use telephone

Shopping

Food preparation

Housekeeping

Laundry

Mode of transportation

Responsibility for own medication

Ability to handle finances

Box 5.3

Mental State

Assessment of mental function is commonly carried out using the Short Portable Mental Status Questionnaire (SPMSQ; Box 5.4) which asks a series of questions and rates the individual's ability, according to a score, to perform the exam. The individual's score indicates their degree of intellectual function. A more detailed assessment, of course, is required before a definitive

---

Short Portable Mental Status Questionnaire (SPMSQ)
(adapted for United Kingdom)

1   What is the date today?
2   What day of the week is it?
3   What is the name of this place?
4   What is your telephone number/address?
5   How old are you?
6   When were you born?
7   Who is the Prime Minister just now?
8   Who was the previous Prime Minister?
9   What was your mother's maiden name?
10 Subtract 3 from 20 and keep subtracting 3 from each new number, all the way down

0–2 errors	Intact mental function
3–4 errors	Mild intellectual impairment
5–7 errors	Moderate intellectual impairment
8–10 errors	Severe intellectual impairment

Box 5.4

diagnosis of, say, dementia can be made (Pfieffer, 1975).

Social Function

Social functioning can be measured using a tool such as the Older Adult Resources and Services (OARS) Social Resource Scale (Duke University, 1978; Box 5.5). This particular scale asks a wide range of questions about the individual's social network and social support and rates them on a 6-point scale. The position on the scale is determined by the person carrying out the assessment making a judgement, from the responses to the questions in the scale, about which point on the scale best describes the individual. Each point is descriptive and has a number of criteria.

THE OUTCOME OF ASSESSMENT

Assessment and planning in relation to an elderly person is not merely an information-gathering exercise followed by recommendations. The process should be followed by action designed to improve the care of the elderly person. At any stage in the assessment procedure, the process may stop if it is felt that appropriate action can be taken at that level in the process. In other words, the fact that an elderly person is being assessed does not mean that they will necessarily come into contact with the geriatric services, nor does it mean that they will inevitably be admitted to hospital.

If a family notices problems with an elderly relative and bring this to the attention of the person's general practitioner then it may well be possible for the general

Possible ratings from the Older Adult Resources and Services (OARS) Social Resource Scale

Excellent social resources
Social relationships are very satisfying and extensive, and at least one person would take care of client indefinitely

Good social resources
Social relationships are fairly satisfying and adequate, and at least one person would take care of client indefinitely *or* social relationships are very satisfying and extensive, and only short-term help is available

Mildly socially impaired
Social relationships are unsatisfactory, of poor quality and few, but at least one person would take care of client indefinitely *or* social relationships are fairly satisfactory and adequate, and only short-term help is available

Moderately socially impaired
Social relationships are unsatisfactory, of poor quality and few, and only short-term care is available *or* social relationships are at least adequate or satisfactory, but help would only be available now and then

Severely socially impaired
Social relationships are unsatisfactory, of poor quality and few, and help would be available now and then *or* social relationships are at least satisfactory or adequate, but help is not available even now and then

Totally socially impaired
Social relationships are unsatisfactory, of poor quality and few, and help is not available even now and then

Box 5.5

practitioner to make arrangements through the Primary Health Care Team—general practitioner, district nurse and, increasingly, the practice nurse—to institute a programme of support for the person. If further referral is necessary, to the geriatrician, health visitor, social worker or the 'therapists' outlined above, then these workers may be able to institute a programme of care whereby the elderly person can remain at home for as long as possible.

It may be necessary, however, for an elderly person to be admitted to an assessment ward for an inpatient assessment. This, again, does not necessarily mean that they will remain in hospital care; there are many options and these may include returning home with increased social and nursing support, returning home with regular visits to the local day hospital or day centre and also having periodic respite care. It may also be necessary to admit the person for rehabilitative care (to be discussed later) or even directly into long-term care. The possibilities for long-term care include residential homes (local authority), nursing homes (local authority and private) and continuing care (health service).

Assessment does not stop when the initial process has been carried out. Naturally, it is necessary to assess the elderly person in whatever new environment they have been transferred to or at home, with modifications which have been made to maintain independence. This is particularly the case in rehabilitation where it is necessary to gauge the success of the rehabilitative process.

THE NURSING INPUT

Most of the assessment tools described above are not used routinely by nursing staff, but there is nothing to prevent their use by nurses who have the appropriate experience and training. Specific assessment tools for nurses have, however, been developed (Beyea & Matzo, 1989). In the assessment of an elderly person in the community, it is quite possible that a district nurse may use some of these tools but their use by other nurses will depend upon their involvement in the assessment process. This does not mean, however, that these tools have no relevance to nursing staff. If the medical records for an individual contain the details of various measurements which have been performed in the course of an assessment, then the nursing staff have invaluable information which can be included in their own assessment if that elderly person requires nursing care. Specific assessment, for the purposes of nursing care, will be discussed in the chapter on *Continuing Care* (Chapter 7).

As already described, the nurse plays a pivotal role in the process of assessment, and different nursing specialists (e.g. district nurses and health visitors) have an input at different points. The nurse working in a ward that admits older people specifically for the purpose of assessment has to be knowledgeable about the part played by all the members of the assessment team and must also understand the tools and scales which they use. Making the process of being assessed as smooth as possible for the elderly person is an important function of the nurse and this can be achieved by helping to coordinate the activities of the different assessment team members. The nurse also has a unique insight into the abilities of the elderly person in their care and can also gauge how the individual elderly person is coping. The older person may need encouragement to continue with the process or, on the other hand, the assessment team may have to wait until the person is ready to carry on. These judgements will mainly rest with the nursing staff who are caring for the elderly person.

Assessment is not carried out in isolation from the nursing care that a person may require for existing problems. While an assessment is being carried out, the elderly person will need care that prevents deterioration in their condition and prevents any complications (e.g. pressure sores and incontinence) that are not already present but may arise from their condition.

CONCLUSION

The process of assessment is carried out by a team, the membership of which is fairly flexible but which includes certain key members. Assessment is carried out using validated tools, some example of which are given in this chapter. These tools give the relevant members of the assessment team an insight into the functional capacity of the individual elderly person and also give them the basis of a plan for further action—return to the community with appropriate support, admission to long-term care or rehabilitation. The role of the nurse in the assessment team is not as well defined as that of some of the other members but is of great importance in liaising between different specialists and in establishing a relationship with the elderly person such that their experience of the assessment process can be gauged and even regulated according to their abilities. This is quite apart from any nursing assessment (to be discussed in Chapter 7, on *Continuing Care*) and necessary nursing care. The next chapter considers one of the outcomes of the assessment process, namely *Rehabilitation*.

REFERENCES

Beyea S & Matzo M (1989) Assessing elders using the functional health pattern assessment model. *Nurse Educator* **14**(5):32–37.

Duke University Centre for the Study of Ageing and Human Development (1978) *Multidimensional functional assessment: The OARS methodology*. Duke University Press, Durham.

Granger CV, Albrecht GL & Hamilton BB (1979) Outcome of comprehensive medical rehabilitation: measures of PULSES profile and Barthel index. *Archives of Physical Medicine* **60**:145–154.

Katz S & Akpom A (1976) A measure of primary sociobiological functions. *International Journal of Health Services* **6**(3):493–507.

Lawton HP & Brody EM (1969) Assessment of older people: self-maintaining and instrumental activities of daily living. *Gerontologist* 9:179–186.

Pfieffer E (1975) A short portable mental status questionnaire for the assessment of organic brain deficit in elderly patients. *Journal of the American Geriatrics Society* **23**:433–441.

BIBLIOGRAPHY

Lekan-Rutledge D (1988) Functional Assessment. In Matteson MA & McConnel ES (eds) *Gerontological Nursing Concepts and Practice*. WB Saunders, Philadelphia, pp. 57–92.

A comprehensive chapter on the subject which gives examples of many of the rating scales used in this area of work and referred to in the present text. Deals specifically, also, with nursing assessment.

Royal College of Nursing (1990) *Guidelines for the Assessment of Elderly People*. RCN, London.

A good summary of the areas which require assessment; written in response to nurses enquiries to the RCN about the subject.

Sehy YA & Williams MP (1991) Functional assessment. In Chenitz WC, Stone JT & Salisbury SA (eds) *Clinical Gerontological Nursing*. WB Saunders, Philadelphia, pp. 119–180.

A very concise chapter on the subject, which is included in a section of this textbook entitled Assessment of the Older Client, *which contains four other chapters on physical and cognitive assessment. This chapter has, as an appendix, the questionnaire for the OARS scale reproduced in full.*

Shaw MW (1984) Assessment. In Shaw MW (ed.) *The Challenge of Ageing*. Churchill Livingstone, Melbourne, pp. 76–83.

An excellent chapter on the multidisciplinary approach to assessment.

Chapter 6
Rehabilitation

One possible outcome of assessment of an elderly person might be a programme of rehabilitation, and it is logical that this chapter follows the one on *Assessment*. The functions of assessment and rehabilitation with older people are often combined under one roof or even in the same ward—an assessment/rehabilitation ward. This makes good sense because it means that a formal programme of rehabilitation can begin as soon as assessment has been made, without any delay to the process, with the inevitable inconvenience to the patient of being transferred to another ward or hospital. In other words, the process of assessment actually continues after rehabilitation has started.

It is clear, therefore, that there are wards which see their function as being primarily a rehabilitative one. This does not mean that rehabilitation is, or necessarily should be, carried out exclusively in wards dedicated to that purpose. Nurses in all environments—acute as well as care of the elderly—should be aware of the concept of rehabilitation and the basic premise that rehabilitation of an elderly person should begin as early as possible after problems have been identified. Preferably, rehabilitation should begin on the first day of the development of a disability. This is particularly true of acute disability such as cerebrovascular accident.

Rehabilitation is often described as a philosophy rather than a technique. This is the case because its proponents and practitioners seek to engender an attitude in health-care practitioners which looks beyond the immediate problems of a disabled or impaired elderly person in order to seek out the real causes of disability, be they physical, emotional or social. Merely looking at the physical problems of an older person, such as an amputation, will not lead to good rehabilitative practice. Some elderly people cope well after an amputation and some do not. Likewise, some elderly people respond well to programmes of rehabilitation while some do not, and attempting to understand these differences in potential for rehabilitation lies at the heart of the practice of rehabilitation and research into this subject.

REHABILITATION DEFINED

Rehabilitation can be usefully defined as 'the restoration of the handicapped individual to the fullest physical, mental, social, vocational and economic usefulness of which he is capable' (Williams, 1984), the aim being 'to restore individuals to their former functional and environmental status, or alternatively, to maintain or maximize remaining function'.

While it is perfectly possible to measure the progress of rehabilitation in an individual, it is very difficult to compare techniques or procedures within rehabilitation. It is hard to distinguish, in any individual, between spontaneous recovery and recovery resulting from rehabilitation. This is not an argument against rehabilitation, however, it merely emphasizes the individual nature of each elderly person's response to disability. It is important that practitioners in this area of work do not see old age itself as a disability, but rather see it as another factor that needs to be accounted for in planning a programme of rehabilitation for an individual.

THE REHABILITATION TEAM

It is quite natural that the rehabilitation team bears a remarkable similarity to the assessment team since many of the specialists who were involved in the assessment process will also be involved in the process of rehabilitation (Storrs, 1985). Depending purely upon local resources and arrangements, it may well be the case that they are one and the same team. This will, of course, be the case where there are units which carry out both assessment and rehabilitation. In some areas, however, assessment and rehabilitation will be carried out by different teams and, in some areas, the facilities for rehabilitation may be scarce and the task of rehabilitation will fall upon non-specialized teams. For this reason, as mentioned earlier practitioners in all areas should be aware of the philosophy and practice of rehabilitation.

Where a person has passed through an assessment process and has been considered suitable for rehabilitation, the leader of the rehabilitation team will be the geriatric physician responsible for the care of that individual. The geriatrician will be responsible for placing the person in a suitable unit, for activating the various specialists who might be involved in the process of rehabilitation and for coordinating that process. Ultimately, in consultation with all of the specialists involved in the rehabilitation process, the consultant geriatrician will be responsible for deciding when the process has been completed or taken as far as possible.

Purpose of Rehabilitation

Whatever the combination of factors leading to disability in an elderly person, the main purpose of the process of rehabilitation is to restore and promote physical function, and for these reasons the 'therapists' play an important role. Working from an assessment of physical function the physiotherapist will work to encourage as full as possible the use of limbs, principally the lower limbs, in order that the elderly person can walk and transfer. In addition, the physiotherapist may recommend that an aid, such as a walking stick, may be required in order to promote maximum independence in an elderly person.

The Therapists

The work of the physiotherapist is closely related to that of the occupational therapist who will teach the patient how to be as independent as possible in the activities of daily living. This may only require training programmes to help the person to cope with disability but it may also be the case that personal aids are required or that some adaptations are required in the person's accommodation. Programmes of occupational therapy which involve activities such as making baskets and playing games are not, principally, designed to 'occupy' the person, rather, these activities are designed to improve and maintain manual dexterity and to thereby help in the process of rehabilitation. In the case of patients who have had cerebrovascular accidents that have diminished their ability to chew, swallow and communicate, then the speech therapist will be involved.

The Social Workers

The social worker will be involved at all stages of the rehabilitative process in order to ensure that the elderly person's financial affairs are kept in order and that, for instance, a spouse or other dependant, is managing at home. It may also be possible for the social worker to arrange financial help in order that relatives can visit the person in hospital. This is very important from the psychological point of view, as rehabilitation of an older person will be very hard if they become depressed and thereby lose motivation. If the occupational therapist recommends that some adaptation of the home of the disabled elderly person is required, then it will be through the services of the social worker that this work will be carried out if the elderly person cannot afford to pay for the work.

THE ROLE OF THE NURSE

Last, but by no means least, in the present discussion is the role of the nurse in the process of rehabilitation. While nurses may, indeed, specialize in the work of rehabilitation, they are not specialists in the sense that the therapists described above are specialists. Rather, nurses 'treat the human responses of individuals and groups to actual or potential disability that interrupts or alters function and life satisfaction. The goal of the rehabilitation nurse is to assist the individual or group in the restoration and maintenance of maximum health' (Mumma, 1987). Nevertheless, it can easily be seen that the nurse, perhaps, plays the most important role in the process of rehabilitation. If an elderly person has been admitted to hospital for rehabilitation then nursing staff will be with that person 24 hours a day. For this reason, the nurse needs to ensure that there is continuity in the process of rehabilitation for that individual (Gibbon & Thomson, 1992). The important role of the nurse in rehabilitation has been demonstrated in a study where nurses were responsible for determining the need for therapeutic interventions against a control group (Boyer et al., 1986)

Maintaining Continuity

Continuity is not just a matter of ensuring that the elderly person attends various sessions with specialists; it involves much more. It is essential that there is no conflict between the aims of the therapists for an individual person and the nursing care which is carried out on the ward. While nurses may not be specialists in this area of work, they need to understand the work of several different specialists in order to fulfil this function of ensuring continuity. A basic prerequisite is a system of care planning into which the assessment details and the rehabilitation programme for the individuals in their care can be incorporated. If, for example, the aim of the physiotherapist is to have an elderly person walking independently and one of the objectives on the way to that aim is walking with the aid of one stick for a short time, the nurse should be aware which stage of the rehabilitation process the patient has reached, in order to implement the appropriate level of assistance on the ward. This is very important, as attempting to hasten the process could lead to a loss of confidence by the disabled person. On the other hand, if the nurse gives too much assistance, the process of rehabilitation could be undermined. Nurses need to give these matters very serious consideration because, despite the fact that they may not not be carrying out the assessments and dictating the programme of mobilization, they are responsible for implementing much of their programme through 'informal' physiotherapy. Opportunities to implement this should not be missed, and each trip to the toilet or walk to the day room should be seen as an opportunity to encourage an older person in their rehabilitation.

Likewise, with occupational therapy, the therapist will assess the person's ability and suggest a programme, for example, for dressing and the nurse should be familiar with that programme, in order that the elderly person can be given the appropriate level of assistance and not have too much or too little done for them by the nurse. Again, the nurse will be mainly responsible for implementing the programme of occupational therapy.

Liaison with the Therapists

Nurses have much to learn from the therapists and every opportunity should be taken to tap these valuable sources of expert knowledge about the rehabilitation process. Specific details of the programme for an individual should be sought and advice should be taken on, for example, how one nurse is to walk a patient who is learning to walk after a cerebrovascular accident. Close liaison between the therapists and the nursing staff will engender confidence in the disabled elderly person and will ensure that there is no difference in practice between departments.

The nurse, rather than the therapist, is most likely to be the person who comes into contact with relatives of the disabled person, and a nurse who is well informed about the rehabilitation process will be better able to explain the therapy that the elderly person is receiving and what kind of progress they are making. If someone is being discharged after a course of rehabilitation then it is up to the nurse to ensure that the relatives, or anyone who will be involved with the care of the disabled person at home, is aware of their abilities and also their limitations.

THE PROCESS OF REHABILITATION

One of the underlying principles of rehabilitation is prevention. Prevention is the maintenance of function or the prevention of deterioration in an organ or system that is not primarily involved in the condition of the patient. The remainder of the work of rehabilitation is properly called restoration, which is involved with the process of bringing individuals to their highest potential. A programme of rehabilitation will be of no value if fundamental preventative nursing and therapy are not carried out. The fact that a person is undergoing rehabilitation does not mean that these aspects of care can be ignored. Attention should be paid to the areas in Box 6.1. Nurses should pay attention to correct lifting procedures with older people. There is no point; for example, in rehabilitating a

---

Preventative nursing aspects of rehabilitation

Physical
Pressure sores, venous stasis, immobility of joints, contraction of muscles, constipation, incontinence

Psychological
Boredom, depression

Box 6.1

person to walk independently if, through poor lifting techniques, they have developed painful shoulders.

Realistic Goal Setting

Assessment is obviously fundamental to the process of rehabilitation; the process of assessment has been discussed in the previous chapter. On the basis of the assessment, the main problems for an individual can be identified and a programme of rehabilitation can be planned.

Integral to the programme of rehabilitation is that of goal setting. Goals are necessary in order that the members of the rehabilitation team can gauge the effectiveness of their programme. Goals need to be sufficiently high in order to offer the disabled person some benefit from the rehabilitation programme but, at the same time, they must be realistic and achievable otherwise the disabled person and the rehabilitation team will become demoralized. Good goal setting is, therefore, very important. In the process of rehabilitation it is far better at some point to be able, on the basis of goals already achieved, to increase the goals rather than having to decrease the goals as a result of the disabled person's inability to reach the goals which have already been set. The best goals are those which have been drawn up with the involvement and consent of the disabled elderly person.

The programme of rehabilitation must be implemented consistently with all members of the team—with the disabled person being at the centre of the process—fully informed of the aims and objectives for the individual. The framework of the team has been described earlier, and this framework needs to be used in order for the implementation to work. It is beyond the scope of this book to give a detailed account of the implementation of a programme of rehabilitation. The purpose, rather, is to describe the basic principles and to show nurses how they can play an effective role.

EVALUATING REHABILITATION

In order to gauge the effectiveness of the rehabilitation programme it is necessary to evaluate periodically. The frequency of the evaluation will depend upon the individual disabled person, the extent of their disability and the goals which have been set. The basis of the evaluation will be the goals which have been set and whether or not the individual is being enabled to achieve them. Evaluation is best carried out by the therapists who carried out the initial assessment and who set the goals of the rehabilitation programme. Anecdotal reporting on an individual's ability should not be too heavily relied upon. Instead, detailed functional assessment should be carried out and the details of progress recorded and reported back to the whole rehabilitation team with any changes which have been made to the programme on the basis of the evaluation.

Measurement in Rehabilitation

Measurement, in the process of rehabilitation, begins with estimating the extent of disability and also using functional assessment. This can be achieved using agreed criteria.

Disability has already been discussed in Chapter 2, in terms of the World Health Organization definitions of impairment, disability and handicap. These criteria refer to specific abnormalities of structure or function in the body. It is important to assess these in elderly people but, as has been discussed above, rehabilitation is really concerned with how individuals respond to disability and not with the disability itself. Impairment, a disability or handicap are things that the individual will have to learn to live with. Generally they cannot be treated and the rehabilitation process is not aimed at improving these.

Functional Ability

The rehabilitation process is aimed at functional ability, in other words, how the level of disability in an individual adversely influences their ability to function in activities of daily living and also in the instrumental activities of daily living, i.e. socially and even psychologically. For example, a person who is rendered hemiplegic as a result of a stroke may be able to function quite well afterwards if they can be enabled to walk and to cope psychologically with their handicap. Another person may be ashamed to leave their home or even the hospital in this condition, and it is going to be very hard to rehabilitate them. For these reasons, the emphasis in rehabilitation is on functional ability and, for this reason, measurement of functional assessment is vital to the process of rehabilitation. Some of the measurement tools have already been discussed in the previous chapter on assessment and, of course, many of them apply directly to evaluation in the process of rehabilitation. Unlike disability, it is possible with rehabilitation to improve an individual's level of functional ability and, in order not to repeat much of the information in the previous chapter, a convenient way of looking at the process is on a simple 5-point functional rating scale (given in Shaw, 1984; Box 6.2), which looks at movement on a scale from being severely dependent to being completely independent and uses this to assess the individual, to set goals and to evaluate throughout the rehabilitation process.

CONCLUSION

Rehabilitation is a process that is dependent on good nursing care and on good interdisciplinary teamwork. The nurse is mainly responsible for ensuring that deterioration in the condition of the individual does not take place during the process of rehabilitation, as

---

A functional rating scale for rehabilitation

1 **Complete independence**
   Able to live alone as client wishes

2 **Dependent in an adapted environment**
   Able to live alone if special needs are met

3 **Semi-dependent**
   Able to self-care with assistance from another person to perform some activities

4 **Dependent**
   Requires assistance from another person for most activities

5 **Severely dependent**
   Unable to participate in own care at all

Box 6.2

well as for ensuring that there is continuity of restorative care throughout the process. For these reasons, nurses working in this area must have a good understanding of the work of other professionals such as physiotherapists and occupational therapists, to name but two.

The process of rehabilitation is dependent upon good assessment and on the setting of realistic goals for the individual older person who is suitable for rehabilitation. Furthermore, it is essential that there is evaluation during the rehabilitative process in order to ascertain whether the individuals are responding as planned or whether changes are necessary. Realistic goal setting for an individual elderly person participating in a programme of rehabilitation is best achieved by involving the person as much as possible. After all, they are central to the programme.

Nurses working in rehabilitation can be specialists, but all nurses working in any environment with older people need to be aware of the principles involved because the process needs to begin as soon as is realistically possible if good results are to be achieved. Specialist rehabilitation facilities are favoured, but a good dissemination of the philosophy and practice of rehabilitation to the whole of the nursing profession is also desirable.

REFERENCES

Boyer N, Chuang JC & Gniper D (1986) An acute care geriatric unit. *Nursing Management* **17**(5):22–25.

Gibbon B & Thomson A (1992) The role of the nurse in rehabilitation. *Nursing Standard* **6**(36):32–35.

Mumma C (ed.) (1987) *Rehabilitation Nursing: Concepts and Practice*, 2nd Edition. Rehabilitation Nursing Foundation, Evanstown.

Shaw MW (1984) In Shaw MW (ed.) Restorative Care. *The Challenge of Ageing*. Churchill Livingstone, Melbourne, pp. 92–101.

Storrs, AM (1985) Rehabilitation. In *Geriatric Nursing*, 3rd Edition. Baillière Tindall, London, pp. 141–156.

Williams TF (ed.) (1984) *Rehabilitation in the Ageing*. Raven Press, New York.

BIBLIOGRAPHY

Davies S (1990) Nurse-managed care in a rehabilitation ward. *Nursing Times* **86**(38):56.

A short report on the management of rehabilitation by nursing staff, and the possible benefits of better communication and better defined goals for the patient.

Gibbon B & Thomson A (1992) The role of the nurse in rehabilitation. *Nursing Standard* **6**(36):32–35.

A report on work which tries to define the parameters of the work of the nurse in rehabilitation.

Middleton S (1990) Solving an age old problem. *Nursing Times* **86**(17):49–52.

An article on the different needs of elderly people requiring rehabilitation and how this was accommodated in one health authority.

Phipps MA & Kelly-Hayes M (1991) Rehabilitation of older adults. In Baines EM (ed.) *Perspectives on Gerontological Nursing*. Sage, Newbury Park, pp. 357–372.

A research-based chapter which looks at the development of the role of nurses within rehabilitation, the present practice of rehabilitation nursing and what remains to be investigated for the future.

Shaw MW (1984) Restorative care, In Shaw MW (ed.) *The*

Challenge of Ageing. Churchill Livingstone, Melbourne, pp. 92–101.

A very common-sense look at rehabilitation. Emphasizes that rehabilitation can only really be evaluated through functional assessment.

Squires A (1989) *Rehabilitation of the Older Patient. A Handbook for the Multidisciplinary Team.* Croom Helm, London.

Covers the work of the whole multidisciplinary team. Addresses the issue of the key worker and leadership in the rehabilitation team. Clearly written and comprehensive.

Chapter 7
Continuing Care

Continuing care refers to long-term care in a variety of settings, including local authority or private residential homes, private nursing homes and hospital. This chapter will be concerned, primarily, with long-term care in hospital. In total, there are about 350 000 elderly people in continuing care, both nursing and residential (Rooker, 1991). In 1987, there were over 100 000 people in nursing homes and slightly over half of these were in private care (Haywood, 1991). The proportion of elderly people in private care is steadily growing.

It must be said at the outset of this chapter that long-term care could hardly ever be described as the way in which any elderly person would wish to spend their days. This is not, in any way, meant to paint a negative picture of this particular aspect of caring for elderly people. In precisely the same way as no individual would choose to spend time as a patient in the intensive care unit of a general hospital, no individual would choose continuing care because both types of care indicate a very high level of dependency. However, the very fact that it is seen to be necessary, with all of the consequences and attendant problems which it has for the individual, makes this area of care particularly interesting, challenging and rewarding for the nurse. Some of the problems that arise in continuing care are not unique to this setting but they are particularly acute here. For this reason, these problems have received particular attention by nurses working in this area, and nurses in other settings may have much to learn from them.

ADMISSION TO CONTINUING CARE

The decision to admit an elderly person to continuing care is not one that would ever be taken lightly by a geriatric physician. Apart from any other reason, places in continuing care are becoming scarce as the number of elderly people increases and resources are concentrated elsewhere, for example, in the community (see Chapter 4).

Admission to continuing care will be the result of a process which will certainly have involved assessment and, perhaps, rehabilitation. It is to be hoped that, in many cases, an elderly person being admitted to a continuing-care setting in hospital will have already had day-care facilities and even respite admissions to the ward where the admission is made.

The 'end of the road' myth about continuing care should be dispelled at the earliest possible opportunity. In terms of a process of medical and nursing care, the continuing care setting may, indeed, be the final one in a series of admissions. This, of course, raises anxieties in older people and their relatives. However, the 'end of the road' is neither the objective nor the reality of the continuing care of elderly people. Continuing care is meant to be a setting in which the potential of each older person, regardless of how the abilities of the individual have deteriorated through ageing and illness, can be attained.

Admittedly, bad practices have occurred in long-term care settings as they have in all areas of nursing. The physical and psychological stresses, outdated buildings, restricted resources and poor image of nursing elderly people have probably contributed to this (Millard & Roberts, 1991). However, while bad practices need to be highlighted and dealt with, in whatever setting they arise, the standards of care in the nursing of elderly people will only be raised by illuminating good practice and expounding upon sound theory.

ISSUES IN CONTINUING CARE

As intimated earlier, some of the problems of continuing care are not unique to this setting, but they become particularly acute due to the fact that the older person is liable to spend many months and even years in such care. All of the problems of being removed from a familiar environment, which are common to all hospital settings, are present. Lack of privacy and personal space, again common to all hospital settings, are heightened because, unlike in the acute setting, this is not just a temporary phase of a person's life. An end to autonomy and a loss of control over one's life may become apparent and none of this is seen as being desirable by an individual. It is certainly not beneficial.

Institutionalization

There is a distinct set of conditions arising out of these problems which is described as *institutionalization*. The main features of this phenomenon are identified in Box 7.1 (Goffman, 1961). There is no suggestion that such a regime is deliberately enforced on elderly people in continuing care. Rather, it can be appreciated that most of the features in Box 7.1 are the result of the design of many of the institutions in which continuing care of the elderly is carried out. Nevertheless, features of institutionalization can be identified (Box 7.2; King

---

Features of institutionalization

All aspects of life occur in the same place

Each daily living activity occurs with a large number of people

All daily activities are tightly scheduled and occur in orderly sequence

All enforced activities are designed to meet the aims of the institution

---

Box 7.1

et al, 1971) which definitely do result from the way in which care is delivered in continuing-care settings. In order to gauge the extent of institutionalization four so-called dimensions have been identified; these are shown in Box 7.3 (Pincus, 1986). It should be emphasized that institutionalization is not only a feature of long-term care but can equally be a feature of assessment and rehabilitation environments.

Outcome of institutionalization

Depersonalization, providing few personal possessions and limited privacy

Social distance between residents and staff

Block treatment, characterized by queuing and batch processing of activities in orderly sequence

Lack of variation in the daily routine

Box 7.2

Dimensions of institutionalization

Public/private
The ability of the resident to have a private domain
which is not open to public view or use, and which
the institution will not transgress

Structured/unstructured
The degree to which the resident is expected to
conform to rules and discipline, and his/her ability
to make decisions or to have a choice

Resource–sparse/resource–rich
This assesses the degree of the resident to be able
to engage in work or lesser activities

Isolated/integrated
This assesses the opportunity for communication
and reaction with the world outside the home

Box 7.3

It can easily be seen how institutionalization can
'set in' in continuing care of the elderly settings.
Traditionally these have not been designed for the
continuing care of elderly people. Rather they have
often been former 'workhouses' or 'poorhouses', where
an element of correction and improvement was part
of the philosophy of the institution. The very design
of some buildings deliberately includes features such
that maximum observation of residents, with a concomitant minimum of privacy, is ensured. Sleeping
areas and washrooms are often communal and the
buildings are situated away from the bulk of the
population such that residents become isolated from
normal life. In some cases, other types of hospital

wards and even whole hospitals which have outlived their usefulness for acute medicine and surgery or whose functions have ceased, such as former infectious diseases hospitals, have been given over to continuing care of the elderly. Moreover, these hospitals are often under-staffed and suffer from poor resource allocation. The potential therefore exists for a vicious circle to be established whereby the staff themselves become institutionalized and less motivated to deliver care that is not institutional.

Staff

Delivering care in an institutional way may appear, superficially, to have advantages for staff. First, it provides a regime in which everyone from the managers to the auxiliaries feels safe; everyone knows their job from the beginning to the end of a shift and the system can almost run itself. Second, and related to the above, it provides a way of getting the work done; it also gives goals—staff-oriented goals—which can be achieved and, thereby, engender a sense of achievement at the end of the day. None of this is, of course, patient-centred but it can be seen that it is not an easy task for the enlightened nurse to tackle this phenomenon, which may have been the established practice in a ward, a unit or even a hospital, for decades. As examples, it requires much less effort if residents all rise at the same time in the morning, wear clothes which can be taken from a central store, eat their meals in a way which is convenient for the staff and the institution, have personal hygiene attended to on a rota ('bathing-book') basis and spend the majority of their time watching the television.

Buildings

On the other hand, there are many exemplary modern
and purpose-built hospitals which, at least, show fewer
'built-in' institutional features.These include smaller
or even individualized sleeping areas, attractive dining
rooms with flexible mealtimes and plenty of activities
out of the ward area. There are even examples of
old, initially institutional, buildings which have been
suitably adapted for continuing care of the elderly by
partitioning sleeping areas into smaller units, reducing
the number of residents, and making imaginative use
of the space thus created for therapy and recreational
areas. Whatever the setting, however, the challenge is
there for nursing staff and others to provide an
environment and a philosophy of care which is less
institutionalized and more suited to the individuals
who are being cared for.

It is relatively easy to identify the problem of
institutionalization; it can be defined, described,
abhorred and lamented. There is a need, however, for
solutions to this problem, and while all of these may
not be applicable or even possible in every setting, it
is possible to make a start in any environment to
lessen the impact of the institution.

Fighting Institutionalization

Fighting institutionalization initially involves recognizing the features of the problem which have been
outlined. Once the features are recognized then, wherever possible, they should be tackled by overcoming
or eliminating them in some way. This, however,
requires coordinated action and local policies to ensure
that the 'fight' is not just a paper exercise but is

translated into action on behalf of older people in continuing care. This section looks at some specific ways in which the problem can be tackled and thereby translates the 'fight' against institutionalization in general into some specific practical points of action.

The fight against institutionalization begins as soon as the elderly person arrives in the continuing-care setting. One of the foremost weapons is the application of a sound nursing philosophy on the ward, which is expressed in thorough and workable care plans. None of these features should be unique to continuing care of the elderly but it is felt that they are particularly applicable here and, as stated in the introduction to this chapter, there may be much to be learned by nurses in other areas of care.

Philosophy of Care

A good starting point for any area is to draw up a statement of the unit's philosophy, which contains the aims of care and which is common knowledge to all nurses working in that area. In order to achieve this, it is better if the philosophy of care applies to as small an area as possible, i.e. to single-wards, and for this reason it can be composed by all of the nurses in that ward and thereby 'owned' by them. Naturally, any such philosophies require to be ratified by nursing management in order to ensure that they are sound but, once drawn up and ratified, they should be respected. Suitable points for inclusion in any statement of philosophy would be the emphasis on the independence and dignity of the elderly person; the involvement of the family; the rationale for delivery of care; and any realistic statements that engender confidence in the residents and their relatives and help to forge a sense of identity and unity among the nursing staff. Box 7.4 (Awareness Third Age, 1989) shows an example of a general consensus statement on a philosophy of care for elderly people drawn up by a multidisciplinary team.

Organization of Care

Organization of care has received increasing attention in recent years, and one system of care delivery which has been found to be particularly appropriate to continuing care of the elderly is that of primary nursing. Primary nursing is identifiable by a number

---

A multidisciplinary consensus statement

1 Age should not be an influential factor that differentiates care; we believe that elderly people are individuals who have the right to make health care decisions which incorporate personal values and beliefs, respecting and maintaining privacy, dignity, independence, security and confidentiality

2 We believe elderly people should be enabled to develop their full diverse potential, maximizing their capabilities, and acknowledging the concept and right of self-determination within realistic goals

3 We believe that to improve or maintain the quality of life of clients and carers there should be coordination and continuity of care and right of access to all resources

---

Box 7.4

of features (McGuire, 1989; Box 7.5), but it is often the case that it is not implemented to the full in any particular area. In these cases it is usually referred to as modified primary nursing.

The essential outcome of primary nursing is that it moves the delivery of care away from a system which is either routine or simply formulated at the management level in any unit. Qualified nurses (primary nurses) have an allocated group of residents who they are responsible for assessing upon admission and whose care they plan in a systematic fashion. Ideally, the primary nurse should have their own team of staff but it is appreciated that this is rarely achievable. It is important, nevertheless, that all of the staff are aware of who the primary nurses are for particular residents and refer to them for any proposed changes in care. Under these circumstances all other staff become 'associate nurses' to the primary nurse with respect to a particular group of residents.

The potential benefits of the implementation of primary nursing are that it devolves responsibility for care to qualified nurses and allows for a more intimate and ongoing relationship to be developed between primary nurses and their group of residents. In this way, it also allows for greater accountability by individual nurses in continuing care. Residents and relatives should be aware of who their primary nurse is and should see them as their first point of contact within the unit for any problems regarding care.

The Nursing Process

The nursing process is almost ubiquitous in British nursing today and its basic elements of assessment, planning, implementation and evaluation (leading to

Key features of primary nursing

1 Each resident is allocated to a named nurse, the primary nurse, who is responsible for and accountable to that resident for the whole period of his or her care

2 The primary nurse has 24-hour responsibility for that resident

3 The primary nurse is responsible for carrying out the nursing assessment of that resident, planning the nursing care to be given and evaluating the outcome of the nursing care given

4 Planning and evaluation of nursing care is carried out in collaboration with medical staff and in conjunction with the resident and resident's relatives (where possible)

5 The primary nurse is responsible for coordinating the contribution of other health care professionals to the care of the resident

6 A major part of the direct personal care given to that resident is given by the primary nurse

7 The primary nurse is assisted in the direct care of a resident by an associate nurse who takes over the giving of care when the primary nurse is not on duty. The associate nurse carries out the care as detailed in the care plan and must consult with the primary nurse before any major changes are made. A nurse may act in the capacity of associate nurse in relation to some residents and as a primary nurse in relation to other residents

8 Where there are learner nurses on the ward, each is assigned to work with a named primary nurse and her residents

Box 7.5

Key features of primary nursing

9 The primary nurse is supported in her role by a clinical nurse specialist (or other senior nurse), to whom she looks for advice in planning and evaluating care and for personal and professional guidance in her work

10 The primary nurse is supported by care assistants and non-nursing staff in the creation of a suitable environment for resident care

---

Box 7.5 continued

onward planning) are obviously very compatible with a system such as primary nursing. Neither primary nursing nor the nursing process on their own are sufficient to implement care in a continuing-care setting, and care is usually achieved by recourse to a conceptual model of nursing. There are many models of nursing. These remain controversial and, on the whole, untested by scientific methods, but they form the basis of much of nursing education and help nurses to establish aims and objectives for care planning.

Two popular models used in continuing care are those of Roper et al (1980) and Orem (1980). Both of these models refer to the activities of living (Box 7.6) (analogous to the activities of daily living) and, in different ways, look at the effect of illness and ageing on the ability of individuals to carry out these activities of living independently, establish deficits, and thereby plan nursing care accordingly. In addition to helping nurses to plan care, such models also help them to make sense of their care. This is especially true in continuing-care settings where nurses are, very often,

---

The activities of living

Maintaining a safe environment

Communicating

Breathing

Eating and drinking

Eliminating waste

Personal cleansing and dressing

Controlling body temperature

Mobilizing

Working and playing

Expressing sexuality

Sleeping

Dying

Box 7.6

not dealing directly with illness nor attempting to facilitate a 'cure' in their patients. Rather, they are aiming to maximize independence, emphasize the dignity of the individual and deliver care which is commensurate with these aims. Needless to say, the adoption of a model of nursing by a continuing-care unit can help in drawing up an appropriate philosophy of care.

Assessment for Continuing Care

Whatever the philosophy, system or model of care adopted by a unit, it is imperative that a suitable system of documentation is also used which allows full expression of all of the features of the way in which care is delivered. It also needs to be used and understood by all of the nurses on the unit, and should allow for aims and objectives to be both stated and periodically evaluated. The adoption of those models of nursing which incorporate the activities of daily living is particularly suitable in any care of the elderly setting because they use the same 'language' as many of the assessment tools used by the assessment and rehabilitation teams. This provides the opportunity for the nurse who is making the initial assessment of an elderly person, upon admission to a care of the elderly unit, to base that assessment, at least in part, upon the work of other members of the multidisciplinary team. Furthermore, it allows for ongoing assessment of individuals to be made, in terms of their changing needs for nursing and multidisciplinary care, which can be compared with their needs on admission. It should be emphasized that, while the multidisciplinary team may not be as evident in continuing care as it is in assessment and rehabilitation units, this does not mean that it is absent. The input of physiotherapy staff is still very valuable, and the occupational therapist has a role to play in helping to assess some of the ongoing problems, such as feeding and dressing, which residents may have.

Admission Procedure

Given that the elderly person being admitted to continuing care is liable to be there for a considerable time, there is no excuse for the admission procedure, from the nursing perspective, to be rushed. This is not an acute medical situation and the nurse can take time to read the notes that accompany the elderly person on admission—medical notes, including occupational-therapy and physiotherapy assessment, social-work assessments and previous nursing notes from other care settings. Much of the initial care plan for the new resident in continuing care can be based on the previous history. The next step would be to approach the resident and find out how they perceive their needs and to gauge whether they have much insight into the level of care which they require. This should be recorded in the care plan along with any likes, dislikes and other personal preferences which may be expressed.

The Care Plan

It is imperative, however, that the care plan is rapidly evaluated, preferably within a week, in order to establish how well the requirements of the resident have been described. The care plan should be seen as an evolving document and sufficient time should be set aside after admission in order to elicit information from the relatives and others who will know the needs of the elderly person, upon admission, better than the nursing staff. Gradually, by means of the care plan, it will be possible to build up a picture that blends the physical, social, medical and nursing requirements of the new resident to continuing care, which can be used to base a stable pattern of care. Any changes, through evaluation of the care plan, should be the result of changes in the requirements of the resident and not the result of hasty and therefore poor initial care planning.

Clothing

Perhaps no single issue in continuing care more aptly fits the description of being a 'litmus test' for institutionalization than clothing (Davidson, 1989). There are two ends of the spectrum in the clothing issue. At one end, older people are kept out of clothing altogether in continuing care, wearing pyjamas and dressing gowns. Thankfully, this is rarely, if ever, observed today. At the other, more favourable end of the spectrum, residents wear their own clothing and have a sufficient supply of clean clothes in order to be neatly dressed every day. In between these two ends of the spectrum there are a number of unsatisfactory situations which represent different degrees of institutionalization and degrees of dignity and independence for the individual residents. There is no value in dwelling upon the unsatisfactory situations. Instead, we will look briefly at what is required to make a good system of individualized clothing work for all the residents in continuing care, and this single issue illustrates a particularly valuable role which the nurse can play.

Individualized Clothing

The basic prerequisite for an individualized clothing system is an adequate supply of clothes. However, individualization of clothing means that the clothes should belong to specific residents and not simply be taken from a central 'pool'. When a resident is admitted it should be possible to ask relatives to take in those clothes from home which the elderly person normally wore. In order to ensure that the clothing does not become lost, it should be labelled immediately in such a way that it is easily identifiable and such that labels do not become removed in the laundry. It requires considerable liaison by the nurse between domestic, sewing room and laundry staff and relatives to make such a system effective. Obviously, it will not always be possible for residents to wear the same type of clothing which they wore at home. Incontinence, in particular, takes a heavy toll of standard items of clothing. Residents who have been handicapped by cerebrovascular accident and thereby have difficulty with buttons and zip fasteners may need specially adapted clothing in order to be able to dress independently. It should be possible to arrange for residents and relatives to buy such clothing, and nurses can advise on what to buy and offer help in selecting clothes which are to the liking of the individual. Finally, in order for a system of individualized clothing to work, a high level of commitment by the nursing staff is required.

Obviously, there is little that nursing staff can do if they have inherited a badly designed building as a continuing care of the elderly setting. However, nursing staff can be active, within such a setting, to minimize the impact of the environment. Conversely, nursing staff lucky enough to work in a purpose-built and well-equipped continuing-care setting should not be complacent about the possibilities of institutionalization developing.

Television and Music

A television is not a bad thing in continuing care because it is a convenient way of keeping residents up-to-date with current affairs as well as providing an occasional means of entertainment. However, residents should exercise some choice over the programmes which are viewed and should certainly be able to avoid watching the television if they do not want to. The television should not simply be switched on at breakfast time and left on until the last resident has gone to bed. At the very least, it should not be situated such that it is inflicted on all of the residents all of the time. In the same vein, the radio should be tuned in to stations which are appropriate to the population in a continuing-care ward. A constant barrage of pop music may suit the young nursing staff but this must seem like torture to an elderly person who has only ever been interested in classical or jazz music. Music, nevertheless, is a pleasant addition to the environment and this can be achieved by having a selection of tapes of different music from the periods when residents on the ward were young and active. An obvious example of this is wartime music and songs, which will help to trigger memories in many of the residents and may even get them singing together.

Newspapers

Another way of helping residents to keep in touch with events outside the ward is to have a regular supply of newspapers delivered. Often it will be possible for residents to pay for their own copy of a paper in addition to having communal copies. Similarly to the issue of music, the newspapers should be appropriate to the population in the unit and local newspapers will be of particular interest. The influence of the institution is diminished when the world outside the ward or hospital is allowed to penetrate, and this also applies to other possible features such as open visiting, allowing family pets on the ward and the willingness of staff to talk to the patients about events outside the institution.

Voting

It must not be forgotten that residents retain all of their human rights while they are in continuing care and, if they are able to exercise these to the full, they should be encouraged and enabled to do so. A good example of where this can be put into action is at the times of local and general elections. If there is any doubt about an individual's ability to exercise their right to vote then the consultant geriatrician can be asked for an opinion. If the person is able to vote then the possibilities include a proxy vote whereby a nominated person, usually a family member, will vote on behalf of the resident (it would not be appropriate for nurses to undertake this) or a postal vote, which the resident can complete in the unit and have posted to the returning officer. The most suitable solution, however, would be to arrange for the person to visit the polling station and cast their own vote in the normal way, if they are able to leave the ward. Political parties are usually more than willing to help with transport on election days.

Outings

Finally, in this brief consideration of continuing care, there is a need for residents to get out of the unit at regular intervals. Residents will differ in their ability to undertake frequent outings, but it should be possible to find something to suit everyone. There is no reason why some reasonably independent residents cannot maintain contacts with clubs and societies of which they were members before coming into continuing care, and it is often the case that such groups will organize the transport for the elderly person. What is required from the nursing staff is to remember the occasions on which individuals will be going out, helping them to get ready and taking into account any special needs which they may have, such as incontinence. Otherwise, nursing staff should be prepared to organize and accompany residents on trips to local events such as shows and village festivals. A natural event in the life of some elderly people is their visit to church, and it should be quite possible to organize, with the help of the church, a regular attendance at their usual place of worship. Relatives will often ask if their elderly resident can go out for a day trip or even go home for a weekend. Provided that nursing staff are satisfied that the relatives can cope with this and are prepared to give any advice and assistance necessary, then this should be encouraged.

Religious Services

Not every resident will have relatives who are able to take them out and not every resident will be able to get out regularly, so it is necessary, on occasions, for activities to be organized in the unit for the benefit of all of the residents. Religious services are a good example of something which can be held on a regular basis. They not only serve the obvious function of attending to the spiritual needs of those residents with a religious faith but also have consequences for all of the residents. Even those who do not attend the services, if these take place on a Sunday, will be reminded of the day of the week and it will help to give them some orientation in time in a routine that may not otherwise have many such indicators. Nursing staff should establish an open and cooperative relationship with the various ministers of religion who visit the ward and should see the value of the work of these professionals, alongside their own work, in the continuing care of the elderly.

It is not the purpose of this chapter to dwell on nursing problems of elderly people in continuing care. Prevalent problems in continuing care such as incontinence and pressure sores will be dealt with in *Section III*.

CONCLUSION

Continuing care of the elderly represents a real challenge to the ingenuity and imagination of nursing staff. While no setting for the long-term care of elderly people can substitute for home, nurses have the challenge of making life as fulfilling as possible for the residents in continuing care and of lessening and even overcoming the effects of institutionalization. This is possible through the application of sound nursing theory and practice, and by drawing upon as wide a variety of sources as possible, including the individual elderly person, for example their abilities, former occupations and pastimes, likes, dislikes and aspirations. All of the above only represents the humane background against which the very high standard of nursing care, which needs to be delivered to a highly dependent and frail population of older people, is carried out.

REFERENCES

Awareness Third Age (1989) Working group (Ayrshire & Arran Health Board). Multidisciplinary Development of Standards in Care of the Elderly, 24 April 1988.

Davidson L (1989) Time for a change. *Nursing Times* **85**(48): 26–28.

Goffman E (1961) *Asylums*. Doubleday Anchor Books, New York.

Haywood S (1991) Standards of institutional care. In Denham MJ (ed.) *Care of the Long-Stay Elderly Patient*. Chapman & Hall, London, pp. 12–28.

King RD, Raynes NV & Tizard J (1971) *Patterns of Residential Care*. Routledge & Kegan Paul, London.

McGuire J (1989) An approach to evaluating the introduction of primary nursing in an acute medical unit for the elderly. *International Journal of Nursing Studies* **26**(3): 253–260.

Millard P & Roberts A (1991) The elderly in hospital. Old and forgotten? *Nursing Times* **87**(22): 24–28.

Orem DE (1980) *Nursing Concepts of Practice*. McGraw-Hill, New York.

Pincus A (1986) The definition and measurement of the institutional environment in institutions for the aged and its impact on residents. *International Journal of Ageing and Human Development* **1**: 117–126.

Rooker J (1991) *Happy to be Home*. Draft Consultation of Labour's Charter for users of Residential/Nursing Care, Jeff Rooker MP, London.

Roper N, Logan W & Tierney A (1980) *The Elements of Nursing*. Churchill Livingstone, Edinburgh.

BIBLIOGRAPHY

Bowling A & Formby J (1992) Hospital and nursing home care for the elderly in an inner city health district. *Nursing Times* **88**(13): 51–54.

   A 'client's-eye' view of how some elderly people in continuing care would like to be occupied.

Denham MJ (ed.) (1991) *Care of the Long-stay Elderly Patient*, 2nd Edition. Chapman & Hall, London.

One of the chapters from this book has already been referred to in this text. This textbook, edited by an eminent geriatrician, covers many relevant aspects of continuing care.

Royal College of Nursing (1991) *A Scandal Waiting to Happen*. RCN, London.

A report on the unsuitability of various long-term care settings for the clients who are in those settings. A number of recommendations are made, including dual registration (health and social care), increased resources to community nursing and better assessment of elderly people.

Royal College of Physicians/British Geriatrics Society (1992) *High Quality Long-term Care for Elderly People*. Royal College of Physicians, London.

Looks at issues determining the quality of care in long-term settings and gives guidelines for audit of such care.

SECTION III: ASPECTS OF CARE

Chapter 8
Continence and Incontinence

The problem of incontinence (one of the 'four giants')
has already been referred to in chapter 2. The purpose
of the present chapter is to review briefly how
continence is achieved and to look specifically at the
problem of incontinence in some detail and to consider
some aspects of the nursing care of the incontinent
individual.

The achievement of continence in childhood and the
maintenance of continence throughout adult life is the
normal state of affairs. Nurses should bear this in
mind when dealing with incontinence in elderly people
in order that they can handle the people who have
continence problems sensitively. There is no room for
negative and judgemental attitudes towards incontinent
elderly people. To become incontinent means that there
is some underlying problem; people do not choose to
become incontinent, and if the problems can be
identified and then treated it may be possible, through
appropriate nursing intervention, to help an individual
to retain continence. If it proves impossible to resolve
the problems which are causing incontinence then it
is certainly possible, through appropriate nursing
intervention, to minimize and even eliminate many of
the subsequent problems.

Incontinence is often a hidden problem, and it is
difficult to obtain accurate figures for the extent of this
disorder in the general population. Some epidemio-
logical studies have been done, however, and these

show that, generally, more women than men suffer and that most people cope without seeking expert advice. Incontinence is still one of the needlessly 'taboo' subjects among the general population and this is reinforced by the media, which has only recently begun to air the subject. Anomalies exist: it is possible to have frank and open discussion of the sexual routes whereby HIV (human immune deficiency virus) may be transmitted and advertising which encourages 'safe sex', yet the Independent Broadcasting Authority has refused to allow advertising of incontinence products that include the terms 'incontinence' and 'bladder'.

THE DEVELOPMENT OF CONTINENCE

The normal state of affairs for the newborn child, up until the age of about 2 years, is incontinence of both bladder and bowel. Until this age, the necessary neuronal pathways have not been established which enable the child to sense the filling of bladder and bowel and then to suppress the desire to micturate or to defaecate. Parents must compensate by looking after the integrity of the child's skin in order to prevent the breakdown which can result from the prolonged contact of urine or faeces. After this time, considerable efforts are invested by parents in 'potty training' children, so that the ability to sense the desire to eliminate and the ability to suppress this desire are regulated towards social norms, i.e. elimination in the appropriate place and at convenient times. The skills necessary to prevent soiling and for personal hygiene are also instilled. A working definition of continence, therefore, could be 'voluntary urination (or defaecation) at the appropriate time, in the appropriate place and without soiling or wetting' (Brundage, 1988). Many physiological factors are necessary for the maintenance of continence, these are outlined in Box 8.1.

As we go through life, apart from the training in socially acceptable habits which we have received, there are also social and, indeed, legal sanctions which can be brought to bear on the person who inappropriately urinates or defaecates, for example, in public. Incontinence is not normal, therefore, and is not, again in common with the remaining 'giants' of geriatric medicine, an inevitable outcome of old age.

INCONTINENCE

If continence is defined as in the previous section, it is possible to define incontinence as 'involunatry urination (or defaecation) at inappropriate times and places and which causes a social or a hygiene problem' (Watson, 1991). The social aspect included in this definition of incontinence is very important for two reasons. The incontinence suffered by an individual

---

Factors required to maintain continence

Intact central nervous system

Good vision

Intact bladder
  Nerves
  Detrusor

Intact musculoskeletal system

Box 8.1

may not cause them any apparent problem, while it can be an enormous problem for friends and family who have to deal with it. The other social aspect is that incontinence can have adverse consequences for the individual for whom the problem is an acute source of embarrassment and a cause of loss of self-esteem, leading to isolation and depression.

Contributing Factors

The contributory factors towards the development of incontinence are both physiological and psychological. The latter can include depression and apathy, which can be sufficiently severe to overcome the normal desire to remain continent. Some psychiatric conditions and organic brain failure such as dementia can also be the underlying cause of incontinence. Physiological and anatomical factors can include damage to the spinal cord which destroys the normal mechanisms for sensing bladder filling and suppression of desire to micturate. Poor vision, urinary tract infection and certain medications such as diuretics are also associated with incontinence. In addition to factors such as childbirth in women and prostatism in men, direct damage to the bladder by trauma or surgery can lead to incontinence.

Causes of Incontinence

There are a number of reasons why incontinence can occur, given all of the above factors and clinical correlates. The prime reason in older people is described as an 'unstable bladder'. Some neurological impairment is present, such that the person cannot effectively prevent contractions of the bladder muscle (the detrusor), and this may be compounded by other problems such as immobility or confusion. The urge to micturate comes on very quickly and the person cannot reach the toilet, leading to incontinence. The same may happen while the person is asleep.

In women, an incompetent sphincter at the outlet to the bladder is often caused by multiple childbirth leading to an inability to prevent urine flowing out of the bladder during periods of increased pressure in the bladder. These include factors that increase intra-abdominal pressure, such as sneezing, coughing or when taking exercise.

Enlargement of the prostate gland in males is the commonest cause of obstruction of urine outflow from the bladder. This leads to incontinence by the mechanism of overflow. However, this can also be caused in both sexes by obstruction due to constipation and also malignant masses (cancer) in the pelvis. As a result of obstruction, the bladder can completely lose tone, a condition called atonic bladder. The bladder fills up, fails to contract but then overflows, leading to incontinence.

Whatever the cause of incontinence, actual incidences of incontinence occur when the pressure of urine in the bladder overcomes the ability of the internal and external (involuntary and voluntary, respectively) sphincters to retain that urine in the bladder. Nevertheless, despite the variety of causes of incontinence resulting in this simple process, it is possible to categorize incontinence, as has been done by the International Continence Society (Box 8.2).

Psychological Effects

Some of the psychological consequences of urinary incontinence have already been mentioned above. In

Classification of incontinence

Stress incontinence
Raising intra-abdominal pressure, e.g. by sneezing
or during exercise, causes leakage of urine from
the bladder. There is no bladder activity. This type
of incontinence often afflicts women who have had
children

Urge incontinence
Takes place with bladder activity but outflow of
urine from the bladder usually takes place before
the person can get to the toilet. They do not have
any advanced warning of the bladder filling up

Overflow incontinence
This also occurs in the absence of bladder activity
and arises because there is some obstruction to the
outflow of urine from the bladder. Normal
micturition is not possible. Eventually the pressure
of urine in the bladder overcomes the obstruction
and an incontinent episode ensues. This is common
in prostatism and in impacted faecal constipation

Reflex incontinence
The result of central nervous system conditions,
such as dementia, in which the bladder empties
due to the reflex stimulated by filling. The ability to
sense the filling and to inhibit emptying are absent

Functional incontinence
This occurs when there is a limiting factor to
continence, be it spinal, psychiatric or
musculoskeletal

Mixed incontinence
As the name suggests, this can be a combination
of any of the above

Box 8.2

summary it is possible to say that urinary incontinence, particularly if it is severe in terms of frequency of occurrence and volume of urine voided, can literally rule a person's life. If the problem is not treated then it can, ultimately, lead to admission to long-term care as the management becomes too much for the individual and the consequences, such as increased laundry, odours and staining of furniture, bedding and carpets, becomes too much for friends and relatives who have been trying to help.

Physical Effects

The physical consequences of incontinence are mainly concerned with the integument. Frequent contact with urine (and faeces) leads to skin excoriation and breakdown. There is an association between incontinence and the development of pressures sores, though the traditionally held view that incontinence causes pressure sores has never been substantiated.

PROMOTION OF CONTINENCE

The promotion of continence is a logical starting place to begin looking at nursing actions in relation to the elimination of urine. Rather than being a specific individualized therapy, the expression 'promotion of continence' applies to a philosophy of nursing practice which aims to prevent the occurrence of incontinence, when possible, and restore continence in individuals who have reversible incontinence.

Many of the strategies which are employed to fight institutionalization (see chapter 7 on *Continuing Care*) can be viewed in the light of the promotion of continence. Routines which may be superimposed on a person's normal pattern of elimination are seen as being counter to promoting continence. It is therefore preferable to have individualized care plans which take elimination into account. Personal clothing is also part of the philosophy of promotion of continence. Individuals who have a sense of dignity and worth are considered to be less likely to become incontinent. Keeping elderly people physically active, including those with cognitive impairment, has been shown to decrease the incidence of urinary incontinence, in addition to its other benefits.

At the unit level, it is possible to ensure that toilet areas are clearly marked and within easy walking distance of all residents. This might involve seating those residents who are at risk of developing incontinence and who have mobility problems within reasonable reach of the toilets. For example, if they have to walk a distance which they know is going to exhaust them they are less likely to ask for help than if they can be helped over a shorter distance. Of much importance in promotion of continence is making the toilets as pleasant as possible for elderly people to visit. While it may be the duty of domestic staff to attend to the cleaning of toilet areas, it is surely the responsibility of the nurse to ensure that they are clean and free of smell. Also, it is important to ensure that the floors are not wet and that there are ample supplies of toilet paper. In order to ensure privacy, the doors should be lockable (although it should be possible, for reasons of safety, to easily open these from the outside) and, if possible, the toilet area should be pleasantly decorated and well heated.

Finally, promotion of continence encompasses the attitude that incontinence should be considered reversible until clearly shown otherwise. This implies that it is possible to assess patients for the kind of incontinence which is present and, in certain cases, take appropriate action in order to treat it.

ASSESSMENT OF CONTINENCE

In order for a proper assessment of incontinence to be made it is necessary for a medical examination to be carried out. This will involve history taking and obtaining a clear picture of the pattern of incontinence which is present. For the latter it may be necessary for a hospital admission to be made and even for urodynamic studies to be carried out. Nurses should encourage patients with incontinence to have proper assessment of the incontinence made in order that appropriate treatment, if such treatment is possible, can be implemented. However, some elderly people find the idea of having such investigations done unacceptable, and the cost-effectiveness of such studies has been questioned (Ouslander & Kane, 1984). In attempting to arrive at a diagnosis, therefore, the underlying problems such as the major diagnosis of illness, the history taking—which should include the time of onset of the incontinence problem, the circumstances under which incontinence occurs and the frequency and amount of incontinence—and the observation of the incontinent patient, possibly on a hospital ward, should allow the type of incontinence to be classified (Miller, 1990). The classification system used by the International Continence Society has been given earlier in this chapter and it should be possible, on the basis of this classification to draw up an appropriate programme of treatment. This can be aimed either at resolving or lessening the incontinence or at selecting an appropriate system for managing the incontinence.

TREATMENT AND MANAGEMENT

Stress Incontinence

Stress incontinence, whereby urine leaks from the bladder upon raising of intra-abdominal pressure, has been shown to be both preventable and eminently treatable. As previously explained, this type of incontinence is more common in women who have had several children and it is now common practice for this type of incontinence to be prevented by teaching new mothers to perform pelvic floor exercises. These exercises are designed to strengthen the skeletal muscles of the pelvic floor which form the external sphincter of the bladder and, in order to be most effective, they should be taught by a midwife or physiotherapist who has been properly trained. It has also shown that they are effective in treating stress incontinence in older women who may not have had the benefit of doing such exercises in their youth (Wells et al, 1991). A new innovation in techniques for strengthening the pelvic floor muscles is the use of vaginal cones. These require the use of the pelvic floor muscles to keep them in situ.

Urge Incontinence

If a person complains that they begin to pass urine without warning or that they just cannot make it to the toilet once they start to pass urine then it is most likely that urge incontinence is present. The bladder is beginning to contract without warning and the person lacks the ability, through some neurological deficit, to inhibit the contraction of the bladder once it has begun. This type of incontinence can be treated by a combination of drug therapy, which helps the bladder to retain urine, and bladder training, which aims to allow the person to regain control over micturition. Bladder training involves a good assessment of the person's normal pattern of micturition. An attempt is then made to follow this pattern in order that the person achieves continence as a first step, and then to gradually increase the length of time between visits to the toilet in order that the person can go for increasingly longer periods without passing urine. Ultimately, if this is successful, the person can achieve full control of their bladder and micturate at their own convenience instead of having to rush to the toilet whenever micturition begins.

Overflow Incontinence

A person who is suffering from overflow incontinence is most likely to complain that they are constantly dribbling urine. Usually this is only a small amount, but sometimes it can be worse. Overflow incontinence is caused by an obstruction to the outlet of the bladder. It can also be caused if, for example in some cases of diabetes, there is an interruption in the nervous pathway between the brain and the bladder. If this type of incontinence is being caused by an obstruction, then the first step is going to be to relieve the cause of the obstruction. In constipation, this is relatively easily achieved; in the case of prostate enlargement, surgical intervention may be required.

Reflex Incontinence

In reflex incontinence the sufferer has no control over continence and the bladder simply empties on a reflex basis after filling up. It is sometimes only possible to manage this incontinence and methods of management will be discussed below. Reflex incontinence cannot, therefore, be 'cured', but there is evidence to suggest that the frequency of incontinence can be reduced and, thereby, the comfort of the patient increased while reducing the workload of nurses with respect to skin care and changing of clothes. One strategy with incontinent patients in continuing care is that of prompted voiding therapy. This involves regularly asking the patient, at hourly or two-hourly intervals, if they require to pass urine and providing the necessary facilities if they wish to do so.

Functional Incontinence

If a person has an intact bladder and urinary tract and has no neurological impairment which directly effects this but is incontinent due to some other disability which reduces their ability to maintain continence then they are suffering from functional incontinence. For example, a person may be immobile or confined to a wheelchair and therefore unable to move to the toilet or to transfer to and from the toilet seat. A person who is functionally incontinent is still able to maintain continence with help and still has the desire to be continent. It is necessary to provide the opportunities for voiding; if the opportunities are not provided then protracted incontinence can ensue, and this must be avoided at all costs.

IRREVERSIBLE INCONTINENCE

The decision that a person's incontinence has become irreversible is a difficult one to take. It means that it has been decided to manage rather than attempt any longer to treat and thereby reduce or eliminate the incontinence. It means a shift in thinking from one where an effort has been made to improve a person's condition to one where the condition is accepted and purely palliative measures, with respect to the incontinence, are going to be taken in the future. This can be associated with a sense of failure in many nurses, and the accusation that one has moved too quickly to the use of devices for management rather than persevering with treatment is often raised. There is always the apocryphal ward sister who cares for a highly dependent and very frail population of patients and who claims to have no incontinence and to have no use for systems of management who is enlisted in support of continued perseverance. However, this apocryphal sister has yet to publish her methods for achieving such high standards of continence care. It is certainly true that the wholesale management of incontinence without proper assessment is undesirable. Such a measure can encourage incontinence where it may have been possible to provide treatment or alleviation.

There are no particular rules for taking the decision that incontinence is irreversible; each elderly person is an individual and the nurses who care for a person are ideally placed to help in the decision about how long treatment of incontinence should persevere before a system of management is employed. The kind of factors which nurses could take into consideration in deciding to move to management of irreversible incontinence could include a sudden deterioration in the patient's general condition which makes it very difficult or impossible for continence to be maintained. The benefits to the patient of continued and failing efforts at toileting in order to achieve continence should be high on the list of priorities. The patient may be too frail to be moved or may be terminally ill. It should also be observed what continued unprotected incontinence, in the face of efforts to toilet, are doing to an individual's integument. The nurse should ask if it is worth persevering, and failing, when the only outcome is excoriated groins, extra laundry and damaged furniture. Also there are associated problems of odour from unmanaged urinary incontinence, and these can lead to embarrassment and isolation. In summary, the nurse should have some idea of what the patient is capable of and how much further it is acceptable to attempt to achieve continence.

Appliances

If appliances are going to be selected to manage urinary incontinence then nurses need some criteria on which to base their choices. Nurses should have general principles for the use of equipment and should also know what they want to achieve for a patient by using a particular appliance. Good general principles are that the appliance selected should keep the patient's skin dry for a reasonable length of time—in order to protect it from the undesirable effects of urine on the skin— and to prevent the patient's clothing from becoming wet. An appliance should have little, or no, adverse influence on a patient's dignity. In addition, although it will be dependent on the previous two factors, the appliance should prevent odour from developing while in use. The safety of the patient should also be considered and this, as will be explained below, definitely militates in favour of particular appliances. The above are general points to be considered for all patients. When it comes to selecting a particular appliance for an individual, then the specific characteristics of the patient and of the appliances need to be considered.

It is not practical to consider all the available appliances here, but out of a list, by no means exhaustive, which includes a variety of pants, both washable and disposable, with absorbent areas, marsupial pants into which absorbent pads can be inserted, dribble pouches, absorbent pads, diapers, pubic pressure devices, urinary sheaths and indwelling catheters, only absorbent pads, urinary sheaths and indwelling catheters will be considered in detail.

Absorbent Pads

Absorbent pads come in several shapes and sizes. Pads are an attractive proposition for the care of a person who is irreversibly incontinent of urine. They are easy to apply to the patient, easy to change when wet and, on a per unit basis, one of the cheapest ways of managing urinary incontinence. While they can fufil most of the criteria outlined above they can prove to be bulky and therefore noticeable, and for this reason they are not always conducive to dignity in an individual. Perhaps the most important factor about them, and research data are available to support this, is the kind of absorbent material they contain. Traditionally such pads have been manufactured containing cellulose fibres which can absorb urine, and the only difference between different pads containing cellulose lies in the amount of cellulose they contain. Obviously, the greater the amount of cellulose in the pad, the greater the amount of urine which they can absorb, but this brings an additional problem of greater bulk both when the pad is dry and especially when it is wet. One way in which absorbent pads have been improved by the manufacturers is by the incorporation of super-absorbent gels into the pads, sometimes in conjunction with cellulose fibres, and these gels can absorb many times their own volume of urine and several times more volumes of urine per volume of cellulose. Research shows that these super-absorbent gels do improve the performance of pads and, while they add to the unit cost of the pads, they increase the cost-effectiveness of using pads and reduce the number of pad changes required for individual patients. (Buchan & Watson, 1991).

Urinary Sheaths

To date, absorbent pads are really the only safe method of managing urinary incontinence in women. Alternative, drainage, devices have been designed for women, but for anatomical reasons these are less suitable for women. Men, on the other hand, have at their disposal a variety of drainage devices and, while these have received unfavourable reports in the past, it is now becoming clear that they are a very valuable method of managing urinary incontinence in some males. In contrast to absorbent pads, which sometimes conflict with dignity, a drainage device can be worn very discreetly. One of the commonest of these devices is the urinary sheath, and this comes in variety of styles. There is evidence to suggest that, from the many styles available, the ones which use internal adhesion are easier to fit, provided that the person is not allergic to the adhesive. One of the reasons why urinary sheaths are sometimes not successful is that they are fitted to the wrong patients. In order for patients to successfully use a urinary sheath they must fulfil several criteria; they should not be too obese or have a retracted penis or any herniation in the groin area; they should not be so agitated that they will simply remove the sheath once it is applied; and they should be assessed for their suitability as an individual for use of a urinary sheath. Some patients, for reasons which have not been adequately investigated, simply cannot keep a urinary sheath in place once it is fitted. Other men have very sensitive skin so that the use of a sheath will cause skin breakdown (Watson & Kuhn, 1990).

Other than the above criteria, it can be said that wherever possible a urinary sheath should be used for the management of irreversible incontinence in males because it is a safe method, provided some basic points of skin hygiene are followed, and it is more dignified than the use of bulky pads. Basic skin hygiene and successful fitting of urinary sheaths involves careful daily washing of the groin area, thorough drying without the use of powders or creams, the appliance of an appropriately sized sheath and the correct fitting of a drainage bag without kinking in the tubing. It is also necessary, for patient comfort, to trim or shave away the pubic hair in the area where the sheath is to be fitted. There is no reason why a urinary sheath cannot be left in place at night, provided that an appropriate drainage bag is used which allows overnight drainage.

Indwelling Catheters

Nurses are generally aware that indwelling catheters are undesirable except in circumstances where they are unavoidable, and this is true for many reasons (Crow et al, 1986). In the management of urinary incontinence, indwelling catheters seem attractive because they are relatively easily fitted; once in place, they offer long-term, total management of urinary incontinence without wetting and odour and in a way which is conducive to the dignity of the patient. However, there are many complications in the use of urinary catheters. Their introduction into the bladder requires strict asepsis and, once they are inserted, they offer an easy route of access for micro-organisms into the bladder and thereby increase the incidence of urinary tract infection in those people who have one inserted. Urinary catheters are liable to blockage due to encrustation, and this can lead either to painful retention of urine or to overflow of urine, bypassing the catheter. With prolonged use they can lead to deformities of the penis and, over time, the size of the bladder decreases significantly. It can be seen, therefore, that the use of indwelling catheters is not to be recommended for the management of urinary incontinence except under certain conditions. These conditions will usually involve an extreme threat to the integument of the patient from urinary incontinence and the failure of all other methods to prevent urine from coming into contact with the skin. For whatever reason an indwelling catheter is inserted, attention must be paid to asepsis in its insertion, prevention of cross infection when emptying and changing drainage bags, and the provision of adequate fluids in order to maintain a flow of dilute urine through the urinary tract. Bladder washouts should be used with great caution, and the introduction of antiseptics such as chlorhexidine into the bladder is not recommended.

CONCLUSION

Urinary incontinence is quite common in elderly people, it is often treatable and is always a problem for the individual sufferer. Nurses should be educated to help in the diagnosis of urinary incontinence and to be ready to offer advice and implement treatment where appropriate. In cases where incontinence proves to be irreversible, it should be possible to manage the problem in such a way that the risks of incontinence are minimized, the dignity of the patient is maintained and no additional threats to the safety of the patient are introduced without due consideration.

REFERENCES

Brundage DJ (1988) Age-related changes in the genitourinary system. In Matteson MA & McConnel ES (eds) *Gerontological Nursing Concepts and Practice*. WB Saunders, Philadelphia pp. 279–289.

Buchan R & Watson R (1991) A nursing trial of absorbent disposable incontinence pads. *Care of the Elderly* **3**(2) 81–84.

Crow R, Chapman RG, Roe B & Wilson J (1986) *A Study of Patients with an Indwelling Urethral Catheter and Related Nursing Practice*. Nursing Practice Research Unit, University of Surrey.

Miller J (1990) Assessing urinary incontinence. *Journal of Gerontological Nursing* **16**(3): 15–19.

Ouslander JG & Kane RL (1984) The costs of urinary incontinence in nursing homes. *Medical Care* **2**(1): 69–79.

Watson R (1991) Incontinence in perspective. *Nursing* **4**(39): 7–10.

Watson R & Kuhn M (1990) The influence of component parts on the performance of urinary sheath systems. *Journal of Advanced Nursing* **15**: 417–422.

Wells TJ, Brink CA, Dionko AC, Wolfe R & Gillis G (1991) Pelvic muscle exercise for stress incontinence in elderly women. *Journal of the American Geriatrics Society* **39**(9): 785–791.

BIBLIOGRAPHY

Cheater FM (1992) Nurses' educational preparation and knowledge concerning continence promotion. *Journal of Advanced Nursing* **17**: 328–338.

A revealing study on the lack of knowledge among nurses of the problem of incontinence.

Creason NS, Grybowski JA, Burgener S, Whippo C, Yeo S & Richardson B (1989) Prompted voiding therapy for urinary incontinence in aged female nursing home residents. *Journal of Advanced Nursing* **14**: 120–126.

This piece of research shows that it is possible to reduce incontinence through appropriate intervention.

Dowd TT (1991) Discovering older women's experience of urinary incontinence. *Research in Nursing & Health* **14**: 179–186.

An interesting insight using the ethnographic research approach.

National Institute of Health Consensus Development Conference (1990) Urinary incontinence in adults. *Journal of the American Geriatrics Society* **38**: 265–272.

A comprehensive survey, from North America, of the problem of incontinence and its management.

Norton C (1991) Eliminating. In Redfern SJ (ed.) *Nursing Elderly People.* Churchill Livingstone, Edinburgh, pp. 185–198.

A very readable chapter from an expert on this subject.

Ouslander JG, Uman G, Urman HN & Rubenstein LZ (1987) Incontinence among nursing home patients: clinical and functional correlates. *Journal of the American Geriatric Society* **35**: 324–330.

Shows that cognitive impairment and drugs are implicated in incontinence.

Palmer MH & McCormick KA (1991) Alterations in elimination: urinary incontinence. In Baines EM (ed.) *Perspectives on Gerontological Nursing*, Sage, Newbury Park, pp. 339–356.

A very good chapter quoting recent research on urinary incontinence.

Specht J, Tunink P, Mass M & Bulechek G (1991) Urinary incontinence. In Maas M, Buckwalter KC & Hardy M (eds) *Nursing Diagnoses and Interventions for the Elderly*. Addison Wesley, Redwood City, pp. 181–204.

A very good account of the problem, giving clear descriptions of the categories of incontinence, possible treatment strategies and assessment.

Stott DJ, Dutton M, Williams BO & MacDonald J (1990) Functional capacity and mental status of elderly people in long-term care in West Glasgow. *Health Bulletin* **48**(1): 17–24.

This study also shows how incontinence increases as you move from less to more dependent areas in care of the elderly.

Thomas TM, Plymat KR, Blannin J & Meade TW (1986) Prevalence of urinary incontinence. *British Medical Journal* **281**: 1243–1245.

A classic UK study of prevalence and epidemiology by an eminent team.

Yu LC (1988) Psychological impact of urinary incontinence. *Nursing Times* **84**(45): 54.

A short report on the psychological aspects of incontinence.

Chapter 9
Skin Care

Skin care is a major consideration for every person who has a reduced capacity to look after themselves either through illness or through disability. The need for attention to skin care increases in older people, however, whether they are in the community or in hospital, and this comes as a result of many different factors.

Skin is a very rapidly growing tissue and the surface layers are continually being replaced from the deeper layers (Hinchliff, 1988). We lose about a gram of skin cells per day, and this process is aided by friction with our clothes and by daily hygiene practices such as showering and bathing. It is possible to see, therefore, that many aspects of old age and disease can have an adverse effect on the skin. Any handicap that reduces general mobility or which restricts the ability of a person to carry out their own hygiene—principally washing and drying—such as reduced movement of the upper limbs, will prevent old skin cells from being shed.This leads to skin which is very dry in appearance and which is flaky. While it probably does no actual harm to the patient, it looks unsightly and lowers self-esteem. An absolute necessity, therefore, for the elderly person who may be impaired or disabled in any way is to have assistance regularly with aspects of personal hygiene which they cannot carry out for themselves and this may often take the form of an assisted bath, or shower, at least weekly.

The real problem, regarding the integument, for elderly people is the possibility of skin breakdown and ulceration, particularly in the form of pressure sores and leg ulcers. Breakdown of the lining of the mouth also poses a particular problem and incontinence has its own associated risks. This chapter will be concerned with pressure sores. A knowledge of the basic preventative measures for pressure sores is assumed, i.e. 2-hourly positional change, and this will not be discussed at length in the chapter.

PRESSURE SORES

Older people have an increased risk of developing pressure sores. This risk is probably only slightly increased by the process of ageing *per se* but is very definitely increased significantly by many of the conditions that are more common in older people.

Intrinsic Factors

The ageing process could increase the risk of pressure sore development by its effects on the skin and on the circulation. With ageing, the regeneration of the skin becomes slower and, consequently, the skin becomes thinner (Tortora & Anagnostakos, 1990). The physical properties of the collagen in skin change with ageing in such a way that skin becomes less elastic, thereby becoming more susceptible to damage through deformation. Reduction in cardiovascular capacity and a less competent arteriovenous system lead to progressively poorer perfusion of the skin. All of these factors, on their own, could lead to an increased risk of pressure sore development, as pressure sores are essentially caused by prolonged deformation of the skin either through direct pressure or by shearing forces which effectively reduce the circulation to the skin. This leads to necrosis (death) of the skin and the development of a pressure sore.

A number of diseases add to this risk, such as diabetes, of which peripheral cardiovascular insufficiency is a feature, and also poor cardiovascular function and respiratory disease, which all have the effect of reducing the blood-oxygen levels in the skin. With respect to pressure sores, these are called the intrinsic factors, and other such factors which contribute to pressure sore development are reduced mobility, malnutrition and peripheral vascular disease. It can be seen that many of these additional intrinsic factors, such as reduced mobility, will compound factors such as lower skin elasticity and reduced skin blood oxygen levels and increase the risk of pressure sore development.

Extrinsic Factors

In addition to the intrinsic factors contributing to pressure sores there are also the extrinsic factors which, in contrast to those factors which result directly from the patient's condition, can be described as things which are 'inflicted' on patients. The extrinsic factors therefore include such things as poor seating, inappropriate positioning, lack of positional change and anything which might contribute to the development of pressure sores.

Poor seating can be taken to mean anything which allows poor posture or slipping and which also leads to areas of high pressure where the patient comes into contact with the seating surface. Poor positioning in seats, but particularly in bed, can contribute towards the development of pressure sores. Sitting up in bed is one of the positions most likely to promote shearing forces at the sacrum because there is very little that can be done to prevent patients from slipping down. Nevertheless, sitting up in bed must be one of the most common positions for patients to adopt, or to be put in to by nursing staff. It is well established that prolonged pressure contributes towards the development of pressure sores, therefore sitting in one position for too long is one of the main extrinsic contributory factors towards the development of pressure sores.

The majority of pressure sores develop in the pelvic region (hip and sacrum) with the heel being the next most common site. The prevalence of pressure sore development increases with age and also, within hospital, there is an increased prevalence in areas where a larger population of elderly people are found. Older people in orthopaedic care seem to be particularly at risk (David et al, 1983). Many surveys have been done showing the prevalence of pressure sores over the years, both in the United Kingdom and abroad. While there are differences in the results of the surveys it certainly cannot be said, even with the heightened awareness that such surveys have generated, that the prevalence of pressure sores is decreasing.

Predicting Pressure Sores

The first attempt to measure the risk of pressure sore development was the Norton scoring system (Norton et al, 1962). This evaluates several intrinsic factors and links the risk of pressure sore development to a particular value derived from the scoring system. The literature on the applicability of the Norton score, and the many other systems which have been developed as 'spin-offs' of the Norton score, is not conclusive on how useful any of them are. Pressure sore risk assessment is always an area of intense research because there are some obvious problems in the use of scoring systems. In the Norton score, for example, a higher risk for the development of pressure sores is ascribed to those patients who remain in bed rather than those who sit in a chair. It is the case, however, that less pressure is developed at the sacrum and the risk of shearing forces are decreased when patients are nursed in bed rather than in a chair. The evidence that this is the case has been available for years, yet the Norton Score continues to be produced in the original format (Watson, 1989a). It is also the case that the contribution of incontinence towards the development of pressure sores has been questioned, but incontinence receives an equal weighting along with other factors in the Norton Score and still appears in other, more recent, variations (Goldstone & Goldstone 1982). Testing of any scoring system raises practical scientific problems and also ethical issues which are beyond the scope of this chapter.

Grading Pressure Sores

While scoring systems can give clues to the practising nurse about the kind of factors to look out for, it is probably better to be aware that all frail elderly people are at risk and, where there is reduced mobility or malnutrition, regular inspection of pressure areas to check for any damage, should be carried out. It is possible to categorize pressure sores according to a variety of grading systems. Some of these are extremely complex, perhaps too complex for regular use in the clinical environment and, in any case, it is not always possible to act appropriately on the information which is gained. The popular and straightforward I–IV grading system of Shea (1975) (Box 9.1) has stood the test of time and its use is strongly recommended here. Combining this system with regular inspection of 'at risk' patients, it is possible to identify grade I sores and grade II sores and to implement appropriate action before the situation deteriorates.

It has been shown that one of the best correlating factors for the prediction of pressure sore development is the level of serum albumin (Holmes et al, 1987). The levels of serum albumin are related to nutritional status and, therefore, it can fairly be said that poor nutritional status, especially protein deficiency, contributes towards pressure sore development. It is probably not realistic or humane to measure serum albumin levels on all elderly people thought to be at risk, but this fact should alert nurses to be aware of poor nutritional status in elderly individuals and to take appropriate measures. It follows that an adequate diet should be part of any regime to treat pressure sores and to prevent the deterioration of an elderly person's skin. Expert advice may have to be sought on the kind of diet that is necessary and on whether supplements need to be included (see Chapter 10).

Grading system for pressure sores

Grade I   Persistent erythema
Grade II   Epidermal damage
Grade III Full skin thickness damage
Grade IV   As for III with formation of a cavity

Box 9.1

Prevention or Treatment?

There is a dichotomy, in the literature, between those measures which are said to be aimed at the 'prevention' of pressure sores as opposed to those which are aimed at 'treatment.' Quite frequently it is stated that 'prevention is better than treatment' and, while this is an admirable sentiment, it often leads to a misleading presentation of the pressure sore problem. This dichotomy is particularly unhelpful in elderly people; prevention and treatment are, at the very least, a continuum and really represent two sides of the same coin (Watson, 1989b).

To illustrate this, consider the case of a person who is elderly, immobile and underweight and therefore thought to be at risk of developing a pressure sore. At the very least, regular positional change, every 2 hours, should be prescribed for such a patient and regular, at least twice daily, inspection made of pressure areas. Is such a course of action prevention or treatment? It may be prevention of the development of a grade I pressure sore but, in order to accomplish this, a form of treatment aimed at the vulnerable pressure areas has been instituted. The dichotomy between prevention and treatment becomes much less clear when regular visual inspection reveals that a grade I pressure sore has developed. This may only be persistent erythema, according to the grading system, but if it was not previously present then it represents a change in the patient's general condition for which measures must be taken.

Are these measures, then, the prevention of the development of a grade II pressure sore or the treatment of a grade I pressure sore? The grade I pressure sore is surely being treated and it may be necessary, in addition to positional change, to use some pressure-distributing surface or to return the patient to bed in order to give more effective relief of pressure. The real danger is that a grade I pressure sore either is not properly recognized or is ignored and not reported and no treatment is prescribed.

Poor Reporting of Pressure Sores

There is, certainly, a reluctance on the part of nurses to report persistent erythematous (reddened) areas as pressure sores due to the association, in the minds of many in health care, of pressure sore development with bad nursing care (Booth, 1992). Apart from the obvious danger to the patient of proceeding to develop a higher grade of pressure sore, this also reinforces the concept that nursing care related to pressure areas and pressure sores is all about prevention and that treatment should be acknowledged as a failure.

There are many more issues which cannot be discussed here but it is important to stress that an over-reliance on scoring systems, combined with an attitude which erroneously classifies treatment as prevention in the care of low-grade pressure sores, may actually endanger patients. It is far better to see certain patients as being at a higher risk of pressure sore development, implementing basic preventative measures—which, of course, continue throughout any course of treatment—providing for regular inspection of pressure areas thought to be in danger of breakdown, and recognizing pressure sores at the earliest possible opportunity. The alternatives are to ignore the potential pressure sores problem until higher grade pressure sores (III and IV) have developed or to provide pressure-distributing surfaces for all patients, whether they are developing low-grade pressure sores or not. This latter approach is simply not cost-effective and represents an unrealistic approach to the problem.

Pressure-distributing Surfaces

A great many pressure-distributing surfaces are available. It is impossible to review them all and some basic principles will be mentioned which can be used as guidelines for purchase and usage. Most of the devices that are effective are expensive and it is worth stating, at this point, that if a patient is not at risk of developing pressure sores then that patient does not require a pressure-relieving surface in bed or in a chair. Obviously, sensible seating for all of the residents of a nursing home or hospital ward which is comfortable and not likely to cause extraordinary pressure, is a prerequisite for any environment in which the frail elderly people are to be cared for. Assessment of the risk of pressure sore development has been discussed above and this assessment should be brought to bear on the choice of support surfaces.

Weight Distribution

The principle of any support surface is that it distributes pressure over as wide as possible an area of the body, thereby reducing the pressure at any one point and reducing the risk of pressure sore development. For instance, in a person who is at risk of developing a pressure sore at the sacrum while sitting up, an effective support surface, on which the person could sit, would be capable of distributing the pressure over the buttocks thereby relieving the pressure at the sacrum. The same principles apply to someone who is in bed and at risk of developing pressure sores at the hip.

People who are confined to wheelchairs are considered to be at high risk of developing pressure sores due to the fact that they are immobile and the fact that wheelchair support surfaces are not very good at distributing pressure. A great deal of the work on developing support surfaces for seating has been done on wheelchairs and some of it is directly applicable to care of the elderly. Foam does not, generally, perform very well, since the sacrum usually comes into contact with the surface below the foam, thereby putting the person at risk of developing a pressure sore. It is to be hoped that rubber ring cushions have been abandoned altogether. These are capable of reducing the pressure at the sacrum to zero but they achieve this by distributing the pressure in a ring around the thighs and buttocks which very effectively restricts the circulation of blood to the sacral area; again, despite the fact that the patient might feel temporarily 'better', this does not decrease their risk of pressure sore development.

Fluid-filled Surfaces

A variety of inflatable, water-filled and gel-filled surfaces have been developed. These are, generally, effective and they are effective by having the ability to conform very well to the shape of the pelvic area which is supporting the patient, and thereby distributing the pressure over as large an area as possible. At the same time, they keep the patient off of the underlying surface of the chair. In this respect, one inflatable surface is thought to be very effective and that is the 'Roho' cushion.

Bed

As mentioned above, the sitting position increases the risk of pressure sore development and, wherever possible, patients who are known to be at risk and who are being treated for a pressure sore, should be nursed in bed. At the very least, bed should be incorporated into their regime of positional change. Standard hospital beds are notoriously poorly designed from the point of view of pressure sore prevention and, when patients are at risk, it is necessary to incorporate some kind of pressure distributing surface in the bed. Towards this end, a variety of mattresses and even specialized beds (such as the Clinitron bed) have been developed.

Some of the mattresses have alternating inflatable cells (the ripple mattress) and, if these are large-cell, as opposed to small-cell, they can be quite effective. The problem with the small-cell ripple mattresses is that the cells, when inflated, produce many areas of high pressure on the body; the large cell mattresses are better at distributing the pressure. The Clinitron bed operates on the basis of alternating inflated large cells.

Water beds have been used but they present problems for administering positional change to the patients; it is very difficult to manoeuvre immobile patients and it is very difficult for patients with any residual ability to change their own position.

A number of mattresses which are not inflatable, but which are filled with fibres, offering good conformation to the shape of the body are available. The key features of these are that they are made up of independent cells, which gives maximum support, they are washable and they maintain their supportive properties over a reasonable number of washes—to be determined by local budgetary restraints. Some of these mattresses offer the facility to remove and replace individual cells.

Sheepskins, while they may be effective at reducing shearing forces in patients who are sitting up in bed (a very bad position from the point of view of pressure sore development) are of little or no value in distributing pressure.

Positional Change

It will have been noticed above that the support surfaces are only used as adjuncts to the basic treatment for patients who are at risk of pressure sore development. That basic treatment is 2-hourly positional change. There has been speculation that 2-hourly care may be too infrequent for some patients but it appears to be effective in the majority of cases, providing a good balance between relief of pressure on the one hand and recovery of tissue which may have been ischaemic, on the other hand. The use of a support surface, therefore, means that 2-hourly positional change must continue and any aids which are available to help in lifting and transferring patients should be used to ensure patient safety and to prevent musculoskeletal damage to members of staff. Lifting slings are of particular value in this respect.

Providing positional change which is adequate to prevent integumental breakdown and which will not psychologically damage a patient requires some imagination and ingenuity on behalf of nursing staff. It should be possible to have the patient sitting up with fellow patients at mealtimes and back in bed at times when the whole ward may be resting. Large bean bags, while they are not popular with every patient, are one way of keeping a person who requires positional change in the dayroom with friends and relatives but providing relief from the harmful effects of remaining too long in the sitting position.

Treatment of Established Pressure Sores

The treatment of pressure sores has, thankfully, been taken from the realm of myth and alchemy into the realm of science. The challenge for nurses is to be aware of the facts about pressure sores and to have a knowledge of such research as is available, in order to apply the appropriate treatments to the pressure sores which do arise in their area of work (Watson, 1989c).

The overlap between prevention and treatment has already been considered and, of course, a prerequisite for any programme of treatment is that those measures which are generally considered to be preventative, are continued. These include 2-hourly positional change, the use of pressure distributing support surfaces and attention to adequate diet and fluid intake.

Grade I Sores

Treatment begins with grade I pressure sores. These may only be areas of persistent erythema but, if they are not treated appropriately, the prolonged occlusion of blood, which leads to the persistent erythema, will cause the superficial layer of skin to become detached, at the very least, and may even lead to the development of a deeper and higher grade of pressure sore. It is quite unnecessary to apply anything to the site of a grade I pressure sore; all that is required to treat this is adequate pressure relief, and the best way to gauge the effectiveness of the pressure relief is the disappearance of the erythema. If, upon application of light pressure to a site of erythema, the area blanches and then refills with blood after the pressure has been removed, then the blood circulation is intact. If this does not happen then the microcirculation has been damaged and a pressure sore will develop unless specific action is taken. The practice of rubbing erythematous areas with the hand, with or without a lotion, is to be strongly discouraged as this has been shown to further damage the microcirculation.

Grade II Sores

A grade II sore has developed if the epidermis, or superficial layer of the skin, has been removed. This can happen due to direct pressure or due to shearing forces; in either case the treatment is the same. As with other types of wound, the principles of occlusion apply whereby semi-permeable dressings are applied in order to lower the oxygen tension on the surface of the wound and encourage angiogenesis (the regeneration of new blood vessels). Semi-permeable dressings also have the benefit of creating a good healing environment for wounds by preventing the loss of beneficial cells such as macrophages from the surface of the wound and also a number of other healing factors. Healing factors include cells and macromolecules which are released during the process of inflammation and which are required for wound healing. A principal benefit of semi-permeable dressings is that they prevent wounds from drying out, which tends to slow down the process of wound healing. For best results, a semi-permeable dressing should be left on for as long as possible. Up to a week is normally achievable with careful application and they can withstand washing and showering.

Grade III Sores

If all of the layers of the skin have been removed then a grade III pressure sore has developed; however, the principles of treatment remain the same. The way of achieving these principles, however, is different. Semi-permeable film dressings are generally not suitable for grade III sores since there tends to be a lot of exudate and this accelerates the removal of the dressing. Some other way of achieving occlusion, moisture and an optimal healing environment at the surface of the wound must be found. This can be achieved using commonly available materials, such as gauze impregnated with liquid paraffin, or more sophisticated and expensive polymer substances. They all work, but there is little evidence to show that more expensive treatments work any better than cheaper ones.

Grade IV Sores

Grade IV sores are sores that have extended down to deeper tissues. Often a cavity will have developed whereby the hole at the surface of the skin is very much smaller than the surface of the wound which is concealed below the skin. The principles of occlusion remain the same, but it is sometimes necessary to pack such wounds with occlusive materials. Light packing of such wounds also prevents the epithelium from closing over the cavity and producing a sinus, in addition to stimulating the proliferation of cells in the healing wound.

Infection

Excessive infection is a problem and it does slow down wound healing (Fox, 1979). However, absolute sterility of a wound is probably not attainable and, if it is attained, it is probably undesirable. The problem of infection stems from necrotic tissue in grade III and IV wounds, and it has to be dealt with by removing the source of the problem, i.e. the necrotic tissue. This can easily be achieved by the use of organic acid desloughing agents and regular immersion bathing. It is not a good policy to try to directly tackle the organisms in an infected pressure sore by means of topical applications such as antiseptics. Most of these are harmful to wound healing and in pressure sores they would normally have to be applied over a long period of time. The above description of treatment has formed the basis of a tried and tested regime for the treatment of pressure sores (Watson, 1989c; Table 9.1).

Measuring Healing

Before leaving the subject of pressure sores it is necessary to say a few words about healing rates. Before it can be clinically gauged whether a treatment is actually working it is necessary to know the original condition of the pressure sore. This can be described in terms of the extent of necrosis or infection of the wound and steps can be taken to improve the wound from these points of view. However, the only thing that will ultimately count is whether a wound decreases in size, and for this it is necessary to measure it. A simple method of measuring has been tested; it involves the measurement, perpendicularly; of two linear dimensions and uses the sum of these dimensions

Table 9.1 Kirklandside regime for the treatment of established pressure sores.

| | | | Grade | |
Condition	I	II	III	IV
Clean	*Regime One*	*Regime one* Semi-occlusive dressing (remain in situ for up to 7 days)	*Regime two* Paraffin gauze* Non-adherent dressing Waterproof tape	*Regime two* Paraffin gauze packing* Non-adherent dressing Waterproof tape
Slough Necrosis Infection	*Regime one* Adequate dietary intake 2-hourly positional change *Regime two* Regime one + daily immersion bath		*Regime two* Desloughing agent Paraffin gauze* Non-adherent dressing Waterproof tape	*Regime two* Desloughing agent Paraffin gauze packing* Non-adherent dressing Waterproof tape

*Change daily.

as an expression of the size of the sore. For cavity wounds it is possible to arrive at the same type of measurement by probing the wound and measuring the dimension below the skin and summing these. In this way, by taking for example weekly measurements, it is possible to follow the healing of a pressure sore.

LEG ULCERS

It is necessary, briefly, to mention leg ulcers in this chapter because they are relevant to the subject of skin care and also because the prevalence of leg ulcers increases with age. Nurses working with older people in hospital and, especially, in the community will frequently have to treat leg ulcers. About 1% of the adult population have leg ulcers, compared with about 3.5% of those aged over 65 years (Ruckley, 1992).

Venous and Arterial Leg Ulcers

The causes of leg ulcers are manifold. The main reason is disease that restricts the venous circulation in the lower leg, accounting for about 70% of leg ulcers (venous ulcers), and disease of the arteries, accounting for about 20% (arterial ulcers). Important aetiological factors are diabetes, obesity, rheumatoid disease and locomotor disease (e.g. Parkinson's disease).

Treatment

Ulcers are usually chronic; one study has shown that more than half of leg ulcers take over 9 months to heal. While the majority of older people with leg ulcers are found in the community and the district nurse probably bears the major responsibility for treatment, it is increasingly the case that specialist leg ulcer clinics are being established in areas where there is a sufficient density of elderly people with leg ulcers. Treatment of leg ulcers is quite a controversial area and it is certainly beyond the scope of this text to examine this in any depth. Compression bandaging is appropriate for most venous leg ulcers but it is certainly not appropriate for arterial leg ulcers (Ruckley, 1992). This should emphasise to the nurse who finds an elderly person with a leg ulcer that a full assessment of the ulcer and the circulation to the lower limb should be made before a course of treatment is prescribed.

CONCLUSION

The possibility of pressure sore development is a fact of life in caring for elderly people. The prevention of pressure sores is wholly desirable but, in some very debilitated individuals, this is not always possible. Grading systems have a place in the prevention of pressure sores, but there is no substitute for regular visual inspection of the pressure areas of patients considered to be at risk. The elderly people who are particularly at risk are those who are immobile and those who are poorly nourished. Prevention of pressure sores can be simply described in terms of imaginative and effective 2-hourly positional change, with the use of support surfaces where necessary.

Treatment of pressure sores begins with the appearance of persistent erythema and, if the skin is damaged to any extent, the principle of occlusion, although achieved in different ways for different grades of sore, is applied. In order to gauge whether pressure sores are healing, it is necessary to make baseline measurements when they are discovered and to continue with regular measurements, in order to see if treatment is being effective.

REFERENCES

Booth B (1992) Pressing problem. *Nursing Times* **88**(31): 19.

David JA, Chapman RG, Chapman EJ & Lockett B (1983) *An Investigation of the Current Methods used in Nursing for the Care of Patients with Established Pressure Sores.* Nursing Practice Research Unit, University of Surrey.

Fox C (1979) Infections as an impairment to wound healing *Journal of Trauma* **19** (suppl): 892–893.

Goldstone LA & Goldstone J (1982) The Norton score: an early warning of pressure sores. *Journal of Advanced Nursing* **7**: 419–426.

Hinchliff S (1988) Innate defences. In Hinchliff S & Montague S (eds) *Physiology for Nursing Practice.* Baillière Tindall, London, pp. 549–578.

Holmes R, Machiano K, Jhangiani SS, Aganval NR & Savino JA (1987) Combating pressure sores—nutritionally. *American Journal of Nursing* **87**: 1301–1303.

Norton D, Exton-Smith AN & McLaren R (1962) *An Investigation of Geriatric Nursing Problems in Hospital.* National Corporation for the Care of Old People, London.

Ruckley CV (1992) Epidemiology of chronic leg ulcers. *Wounds of the Lower Leg*, Tissue Viability Society Autumn Conference, Edinburgh, 15 September 1992.

Shea JD (1975) Pressure sores: classification and management. *Clinical Orthopaedics and Related Research* **112**: 89–100.

Tortora GJ & Anagnostakos NP (1990) The integumentary system. In *Principles of Anatomy and Physiology* 6th Edition. Harper & Row, New York, pp. 119–136.

Watson R (1989a) Sore point. *Geriatric Nursing & Home Care* **9**(4): 26–27.

Watson R (1989b) Pressure sores: their prevention, treatment and management. *Primary Health Care* **7**(5): 4–6.

Watson R (1989c) Pressure sores: a rational approach to treatment. *Nursing Standard* **38**(3): 22–25.

BIBLIOGRAPHY

Bader DL (ed.) (1990) *Pressure Sores—Clinical Practice and Scientific Approach*. Macmillan, London.

A book on the biomechanics of pressure sore development and treatment.

Dyson R (1978) Bedsores—the injuries hospital staff inflict on their patients. *Nursing Mirror* **146**(24): 30–32.

A paper which showed that many of the nursing practices associated with pressure sores, principally rubbing them, actually contributes to the problem.

Exton-Smith AN & Sherwin RW (1961) The prevention of pressure sores: significance of spontaneous bodily movements. *The Lancet*, November 18: 1124–1126.

This classic piece of research using time-lapse photography showed that in immobile patients the risk of pressure sores development was increased.

Livesey B & Simpson G (1989) Hard cost of soft sores. *Health Service Journal* **99**(5): 143–231.

Estimates the annual cost of pressure sores to be several millions of pounds.

Lowthian P (1989) Pressure area care. In Clark JM & Hockey L (eds) *Further Research for Nursing*. Scutari Press, London, pp. 105–112.

This is a very informative chapter, from a recognized expert in pressure sores.

Nyquist R & Hawthorn PJ (1987) The prevalence of pressure sores within an area health authority. *Journal of Advanced Nursing* **12**: 183–187.

The largest study of this nature is the one by David et al (1983), referred to in this chapter, but this more recent study just confirms that the problem is not decreasing.

Shea JD (1975) Pressure sores: classification and management. *Clinical Orthopaedics and Related Research* **112**: 89–100.

This is the original paper which outlines the grading system most commonly in use today.

Stone JT (1991) Pressure sores. In Chenitz WC, Stone JT & Salisbury SA (eds) *Clinical Gerontological Nursing*. WB Saunders, Philadelphia, pp: 247–265.

A comprehensive chapter on the aetiology of pressure sores and their prevention and management.

Torrance C (1983) *Pressure Sores. Aetiology, Treatment and Prevention*. Croom Helm, London.

An excellent book on the subject of pressure sores.

Chapter 10
Nutrition

Elderly people are considered to be at particular risk of developing nutritional problems. There are a number of reasons for this, and the higher prevalence of nutritional problems in older people has been highlighted in a number of surveys (DHSS, 1975; Coates, 1985; Lehman, 1989).

Due to the fact that there are nutritional problems in the community, where the majority of elderly people live, a number of voluntary and social-service organizations exist to ensure that elderly people at home are provided with an adequate daily intake of food. Of particular interest to nurses, however, is the fact that many older people in hospital also suffer from nutritional problems. This has exposed several aspects of the care of elderly people in hospital which may be deficient and which nurses could have a part in improving.

Nurses have always had some education about nutrition in their basic training and it is to be hoped that greater emphasis will be given to this aspect of the care of all patients, but particularly elderly people, in future. Nurses are ideally placed to monitor the nutritional aspects of the care of elderly people and to mobilize a variety of services, such as catering and the more specialized nutritional experts, such as dietitians, towards better nutritional care of their patients.

This chapter will look briefly at some basic nutritional concepts and then examine some of the reasons for the existence of nutritional problems in older people. It will conclude by considering the part that nurses can play in assessing the nutritional needs of elderly people and providing care which ensures that adequate nutrition is obtained.

NUTRITIONAL CONCEPTS

Nutrition is a very complex subject and it would be inappropriate in a book of this nature to cover the different classes of nutrients and the amounts which are necessary for health in great depth. A standard textbook on nutrition or, more specifically, a larger volume on care of the elderly will give details of what the intake of nutrients should be and in what aspects the intakes for older people may differ from those of younger people. The concept of specific recommended daily intakes of nutrients is losing popularity and, instead, guidelines based around ranges of nutrients are being produced (Beaton, 1986). This is so because individuals differ from one another in their daily requirements for nutrients and individuals also differ in their requirements from day to day. The main dietary factors which require attention are shown in Box 10.1.

Nutrient Requirements

In the short term, the most vital nutrient required by all living organisms is water, and without adequate attention to fluid intake all other nutritional care is probably futile. Elderly people, under normal circumstances, require a daily fluid intake of about 1500 ml (Kositzke, 1990).

Key dietary factors

Fluid

Carbohydrate

Fat

Protein

Vitamins

Minerals

Box 10.1

Carbohydrates and Proteins

Daily energy requirements increase from childhood into adulthood and there is no evidence that the need for energy (measured as calories) decreases significantly in old age. Elderly people therefore require a daily energy intake of approximately 2000 kilocalories (kcal) and this is provided by carbohydrate, fat and protein. The principal source of energy in the diet is carbohydrate, although fat and protein have a greater energy content per unit weight than carbohydrate. It is better to obtain as much of the daily calorie intake from carbohydrate as possible and to limit the intake of fat to 30% of total calories. Indigestible carbohydrate (roughage) is the sole source of dietary fibre and the importance of fibre for bowel function is now well recognized, although precise figures for daily intake are hard to obtain. A daily protein intake of about 50–60 g is necessary to maintain body function, and an adequate carbohydrate intake ensures that body protein, principally from muscle, is not broken down to provide energy.

Minerals

The principal minerals required by the body are calcium and iron. Calcium is required for healthy bones, and iron deficiency can lead to anaemia, since iron is required for the synthesis of the blood–oxygen carrying pigment haemoglobin.

Vitamins

A balanced diet will provide adequate levels of vitamins and these can be broadly classified as being either fat or water soluble. The fat soluble vitamins include vitamins A, K and D. Vitamin D is required for the absorption of calcium from the digestive tract and is, therefore, also essential for healthy bones. The water soluble vitamins include the B vitamins and vitamin C. Vitamin B_{12} is also known as the *extrinsic factor* and is required for the formation of healthy red blood cells; deficiency can, therefore, lead to anaemia. Vitamin C is implicated in many body functions, including the formation of red blood cells, and is also required for good wound healing.

Nutritional Status

Rather than recommending specific levels of dietary nutrients it is now considered more useful to assess individuals nutritionally and gain an insight into their nutritional status. Nutritional status is not one single measure or index. Rather, it is a combination of different factors, such as an indication of body weight compared to height; a history of dietary intake with reference to a range of foods and nutrients and taking into consideration a range of health, social and economic factors is required. Assessment of nutritional status tries to ascertain whether the food intake of an individual is sufficient to meet or exceed their needs in order to maintain body composition and function. Detailed nutritional assessment is the realm of the dietitian or trained nurse nutritionist. Nevertheless, nurses are a key source of information in the nutritional assessment of the older people. This can be either through specifically directed assessment criteria by a dietitian or through information obtained from an elderly person, in the community and in hospital, upon admission and in ongoing nursing assessment.

Nutritional Assessment

Nurses need to understand how to interpret nutritional assessment in order to plan care appropriately and provide nutritional support (Collinsworth & Boyle, 1989). Nutritional support is the provision of a balanced diet in terms of energy, protein, minerals and vitamins, in whatever way (for example, as extra food or fluids) is considered appropriate for the individual. Such support may, again, be specifically directed by a dietitian or physician, such as the use of supplements or special diets, or may be nursing care such as helping a patient to make sensible, healthy choices from a menu and providing help with feeding. Supplements are any food or drink which is provided in addition to the 'normal' diet of the individual either at home or in hospital. Once again, in the realm of nutrition, the nurse is involved with the multidisciplinary team; this team can include those already mentioned, such as the dietitian and the physician, but may also include the occupational therapist and the speech therapist.

We will look later in this chapter at how these two other therapists may become involved in nutrition.

THE NUTRITIONAL PROBLEMS OF ELDERLY PEOPLE

That the prevalence of nutritional problems is higher in elderly people has been established by a number of studies. Particular attention has been paid to the nutritional problems of all hospital patients, and this serves to highlight that the problems of older people are particularly acute when admitted to hospital. Factors leading to malnutrition are shown in Box 10.2 (Storrs, 1985).

Malnutrition

Older people have nutritional problems for a number of reasons including the physiological, the pathological and the psychosocial (Box 10.2). Any of these factors may lead to malnutrition in an elderly person but, more commonly, they may conspire to produce very a poor nutritional state which further jeopardizes the health of the individual. All sorts of malnutrition occur in elderly people, but the most common is straightforward protein/calorie malnutrition leading to low body weight and increased susceptibility to skin damage from pressure sores and also to an increased risk of infection.

Protein/calorie malnutrition can be outlined as follows. An inadequate diet, which contains insufficient protein, carbohydrate and fat to sustain proper body function, leads to a breakdown in body protein. This breakdown is principally of muscle protein and it takes

---

Factors leading to malnutrition

Living alone
Lack of incentive to cook

Physical disability
For example arthritis or cerebrovascular accident leading to difficulty with shopping and cooking

Bereavement
Particularly seen in elderly men who have never cooked for themselves

Depression
Leads to loss of appetite

Low income
Inability to buy appropriate foods, increasing use of convenience foods

Disorders of alimentary tract
Includes ill-fitting dentures, ulcers and hiatus hernia

Abuse of Alcohol
Depletes income and provides 'empty' calories, i.e. energy intake with few other nutritional factors

---

Box 10.2

place because the energy requirements of the body are not being met, as a result of insufficient carbohydrate and fat intake. Under these circumstances protein is broken down and used to make glucose by the liver and muscles. The problem of protein breakdown is compounded by an insufficient intake of protein, which means that the protein which is broken down in the muscles is not replaced. As a result, there is a net breakdown of protein. Protein/calorie malnutrition will rarely occur in isolation, however, particularly if it is sustained for a long time, and the reduced food intake or intake of inappropriate food will eventually lead to vitamin and mineral deficiencies.

Outcome of Malnutrition

A typical outcome from prolonged malnutrition in an elderly person will be weakness due to wasted muscles and tiredness due to low energy (in terms of calorific intake) levels. Such a person may be prone to falls or immobility which lead to injury or pressure sores. in a malnourished elderly person bones will be easily broken and wounds such as pressure sores will heal very poorly.

Causes of Malnutrition

It is quite difficult to differentiate between the physiological and pathological changes that lead to malnutrition in elderly people. It is certainly not the case that malnutrition is inevitable in an older person; therefore the physiological consequences of normal ageing probably do not play a large part in malnutrition. There are some physiological changes, however, that may play a part, such as sensory changes leading to reduced ability to smell and taste food. This may lead to a reduced appetite. The gastrointestinal system becomes less efficient with age, but the importance of this and its contribution to malnutrition is not clear. However, in illness, it is easy to see how a factor such as reduced appetite may become acute and lead to malnutrition in situations, for example infection and after injury, where the energy requirements of the elderly person will be increased.

Disease. Chronic conditions such as cerebrovascular disease, arthritis, diabetes and mental disorders all contribute towards malnutrition in elderly people. It does not take much imagination to see how any of these or, quite commonly, a combination of them can lead to malnutrition. Arthritis can lead to immobility, and the consequences may be both an inability to visit the local shops in order to buy provisions and, even if this can be achieved, it may be difficult to prepare food properly. Mental disorders, such as dementia (which will be given special consideration later), may lead to apathy about diet, and if a chronic metabolic condition such as diabetes is present then it becomes very difficult to maintain a stable blood glucose level. Cerebrovascular accident poses a number of problems which are relevant to nutrition. Reduced use of lower limbs leads to immobility, with its attendant problems, and the ability to prepare and eat food may be severely affected by reduced function of upper limbs. More specific to cerebrovascular accident is the problem of dysphagia (reduced ability to swallow), which may lead to severe nutritional problems in addition to increasing risk of aspiration and asphyxiation. These are some of the common problems but the list could be extended.

Psychosocial factors. A similar picture is presented by the psychosocial factors that may lead to malnutrition in older people. Any of the conditions mentioned in the previous paragraph may be present but can be compounded in an elderly person by loneliness, bereavement, poverty and depression. Bereavement is a particular problem in elderly men who may never have cooked for themselves. Another factor which is prevalent in older people is excessive use of alcohol. Alcohol is a good source of calories, but dependence on alcohol leads to an inadequate intake of other nutrients. Moreover, an elderly person who abuses alcohol and who exists on a very low income will be unable to buy sufficient food for an adequate diet. Many elderly people have poor dentition, and many have no teeth (edentulous), and there is some evidence that this leads to poorer nutrition.

Constipation. Constipation is not, strictly speaking, a nutritional disorder. It has many physiological and psychological factors associated with it. However, it may be the case that constipation arises from poor nutrition. The value of fibre in the diet has been mentioned earlier, and it is certainly the case that an inadequate diet will be deficient in fibre. This can arise due to lack of knowledge about the benefits of dietary fibre or as a result of an over-reliance on fibre-poor convenience foods. High-fibre foods require more chewing than lower-fibre food and elderly people with poor dentition may avoid high-fibre foods. Other factors such as immobility, low fluid intake and inadequate toilet facilities may lead to constipation. Psychological factors such as unfamiliarity with sur-roundings and disorientation may lead to constipation when an elderly person is admitted to hospital. Constipation is mentioned here because adequate attention to fibre and fluid intake in an elderly person may help to alleviate the condition (Heaton, 1990).

Obesity. Obesity is a kind of malnutrition, although it may not always be recognized as such. Elderly people may consider it a sign of good health if they are putting on weight. Apart from the obvious adverse consequences on their health, such as high blood pressure, diabetes and heart failure, it is also a sign that proper attention is not being paid to diet (Simopolous, 1985). Again, a number of factors may be operating, such as immobility, poverty and ignorance of the consequences of obesity and how to avoid it. If an elderly person has reduced mobility due to a chronic condition it will follow that their daily calorie requirements will be reduced. They may not, however, compensate for this in their diet and, moreover, there may be a reliance on inexpensive carbohydrate-rich convenience foods. If such a person is admitted to hospital and confined to bed, when mealtimes become the only highlight of the day, then the problem can become particularly acute.

Drugs. Drug therapy can have adverse nutritional consequences and, since the elderly, as a group, are prescribed more drugs than their younger counterparts, it is always worth considering the effect an elderly person's drug regimen may be having on their nutritional status. For the elderly person whose nutritional status is not compromised, drug therapy will usually be tolerated well; but in individuals with a poor nutritional status, drug therapy may lead to further nutritional deterioration. It has been estimated that nearly a third of the drugs being taken by a group of elderly people had nutritional consequences. The most common complication is poor absorption; antibiotics and antacids are examples of drugs, commonly administered to elderly people, that lead to this. Non-steroidal anti-inflammatory drugs can decrease iron absorption leading to anaemia, and corticosteroids

have a range of metabolic and absorptive side-effects
(Rajcevich & Wakefield, 1991).

Dementia

One particular condition, the prevalence of which is
increasing in the elderly, which can have very serious
nutritional consequences is dementia (Watson, 1990).
Demented elderly people have a higher prevalence
of nutritional problems than non-demented elderly
people, both in the community and in hospital. The
reasons for this are not fully understood. Some studies
suggest that there are metabolic consequences of the
condition which lead to this, but it is also the case
that individuals suffering from dementia have problems
with eating, in that they do not always eat the
appropriate foods and can show a tendency towards
both over- and under-eating. In the middle and late
stages of the condition it is almost always the case
that the individual suffering from dementia will have
difficulty with the process of feeding. The outcome for
many demented elderly people is very low body weight
and the attendant risks of developing pressure sores
and being more susceptible to poor wound healing
and infection. The terminal stage of dementia is nearly
always characterized by a complete inability or refusal
to eat even when assistance is rendered by nursing
staff. Elderly people with dementia therefore pose a
particular problem for nurses and the multidisciplinary
team, from the nutritional point of view.

THE ROLE OF THE NURSE IN NUTRITIONAL ASSESSMENT

In the community the nurse will rarely be involved
with nutrition, although the district nurse and, more

commonly, the health visitor, may be involved in giving some advice on diet. The provision of food to elderly people with disabilities in the community is carried out by local authority social services and by voluntary agencies. The specialist nurse nutritionist may be involved with elderly patients who have been discharged from hospital on regimes of enteral or parenteral nutrition, and may work to help the individuals or the relatives to cope with the necessary technology and sterility. In the community, therefore, it will more often be the dietitian who will be involved with elderly people, who will have been referred by the general practitioner. Sometimes these will be people who require quite specialized diets, such as diabetics or coeliacs, but often it will just be people who have been observed to be either over- or underweight and who require some education about their eating habits. With respect to nutritional assessment, the nurse should pay attention to the factors in Box 10.3.

In Hospital

When an elderly person is admitted to hospital, and this chapter will be mainly concerned with elderly people in hospital, the nurse plays a key role in the nutrition of that individual. This role begins with the initial nursing assessment at which time it should be possible for the nurse to ascertain, based on locally agreed guidelines, whether a person has an adequate nutritional status and whether the advice or intervention of a specialist is required.

Importance of Body Weight

The most important indicator of nutritional status that the nurse can use is weight. Three aspects of weight

---

Nursing input for nutritional assessment

Body weight
Related to height using, for example, body mass index or appropriate charts

Weight change
Recent weight loss or increase is of particular interest

Dentition
Does the elderly person wear dentures or are they required? Are existing dentures loose or broken?

Dietary preferences
Personal, cultural and religious aspects of dietary intake

Ability to feed
Can the elderly person transfer food from a plate to the mouth and swallow safely?

Pharmacology
Are any drugs being taken (including self-prescribed medication) which may have adverse nutritional consequences?

Box 10.3

can be investigated, and the first of these is weight upon admission to hospital. The weight should be compared in some way with height, such as in the body mass index which compares the individual's weight in kilograms over height in metres squared (Deurenberg et al, 1989). An index of about 20 is taken to indicate a normal, healthy nutritional status. At this stage in the admission procedure it may be agreed locally to consult the physician, with a view to referral to a dietitian, based on criteria which are considered to indicate malnutrition. If an elderly person does have a very low weight on admission, the nurse can elicit further information either from the individual or from the family about the onset of the weight loss. It is significant whether or not the onset has been slow, i.e. over the past few months or years, compared with rapid onset, i.e. over a few weeks. The latter may indicate a serious condition requiring immediate medical or surgical intervention. After admission, the weight of the person can be continually monitored, for example on a weekly or monthly basis, and any subsequent change can be evaluated and reported as necessary.

Measuring Height

Since it is necessary to measure height relative to weight it is necessary to say something about the measurement of height. This sometimes poses problems in elderly people, because they may have postural problems, such as a stoop or kyphosis, or they may be bedfast, which poses its own problems. Nevertheless, some attempt should be made to measure the height of the elderly person upon admission to hospital. If all else fails then it may be possible to simply ask the elderly person or a relative if the height was known prior to admission. In addition, there are alternative methods of estimating height or of obtaining a measure that can be related to weight for the purposes of nutritional assessment, such as armspan, either from sternum to fingertips or from the fingertips of one arm outstretched to the fingertips of the other (Kwok & Whitelaw, 1991).

Other Aspects

The weight and height (or alternative measurement) should be obtained routinely upon admission of an elderly person to hospital and the weight obtained regularly, on a routine basis, therafter. It is only necessary to measure or estimate the height of an individual once. The responsibility of the nurse for assessment in the realm of nutrition should also include the aim to gain as much information as possible that may have a bearing on present or future nutritional status. Much of this can be incorporated into the care plan for the elderly person. Such information should include likes and dislikes, pattern of eating, and any dietary restriction for medical, cultural or religious reasons. It will be important for the nurse to ask if the person has good dentition, whether or not they have dentures and to observe whether or not these are worn (Geissler & Bates, 1984). Any obvious handicaps, such as paralysis due to cerebrovascular accident or swallowing difficulties, should be recorded and reported. In common with all admission procedures, as much information as possible should be obtained from the individual and this can be supplemented by information obtained from relatives or others who have previously cared for the person.

Dentition

The possibility that some elderly people will have very poor dentition or ill-fitting dentures raises the possibility that they may require the services of a dental practitioner. This introduces other members of the multidisciplinary team, the dental surgeon and the dental hygienist, whose work is relevant to nutrition.

General hospitals will have their own dental department and some care of the elderly hospitals will have facilities that can be used by visiting dental surgeons. In some cases there will be a community dentist who can visit older people both at home and in hospital. The nurse can make referrals directly to the dental practitioner who, in turn, may recommend continued visits by the dental hygienists. Nurses should take the opportunity to learn as much from these specialists as possible. It is essential to know how dentures belonging to an individual elderly person should be cleaned. Not all denture materials will tolerate brushing with toothpaste, and some are not suitable for long soaking in sterilizing fluids. In general, nurses should take very good care of the dentures of elderly people who are unable to look after these by themselves. It should be possible to label dentures, in such a way that this does not show when they are being worn, and it is essential that dentures are cleaned at least daily and are not left to become dry, as this will cause them to become deformed. When not being worn, dentures should be left to soak in clean water (Watson, 1989).

Referrals

The assessment of an elderly person upon admission to hospital is not finished until the information which has been gathered has been properly evaluated and the appropriate referrals, where these are necessary, have been made. Strictly speaking, the nurse cannot directly refer the elderly person to another specialist in the multidisciplinary team, these specialists include the dietitian, the speech therapist and the occupational therapist. Such referrals have to be made through the responsible physician. Referral may be necessary soon after admission due to, for example, low body weight, or it may be necessary during the course of admission, due to an observed poor intake of food or a significant decrease in body weight. The important point from the nursing perspective is to know what is significant, and this will usually be according to locally agreed standards. If such standards do not exist then the nurse should seek guidance from the relevant specialist about when referral should be sought. As examples, it may be the case that the dietitian will want to see an elderly person whose weight changes by 10% relative to their weight upon admission or after the person has been unable to eat the normal hospital diet for a period of 24 hours. For these reasons, there should be provision in the nursing documentation to make the necessary recordings, and nurses should be aware of what to observe for at mealtimes and which patients require observation.

HELPING THE ELDERLY PERSON TO EAT AND DRINK

Apart from those aspects of assessment which have been covered above the responsibility of the nurse, in relation to the nutrition of elderly people, is that of helping the individual to eat and drink. This puts the nurse in a key position relative to all the other services in the hospital such as the catering, the portering and the domestic staff as well as the other members of the multidisciplinary team. The nurse has to be concerned with all aspects of food in hospital, from the provision of adequate choice for each patient, the timing of meals, the environment in which the patients eat and also the specific help which is required by individuals and the provision, at ward level, of any supplements or specialized feeding programmes prescribed by other members of the multidisciplinary team. A summary of nursing practice in relation to helping the elderly person to eat and drink is shown in Box 10.4.

Teamwork

A relationship should be established with the catering department such that constructive feedback can be given on the quality, variety and presentation of food. This can best be achieved by regular meetings between senior ward staff and members of the catering department. In terms of the individual patients, the nurse should play an active part in helping them to select food from the menu which suits their preference, conforms to any dietary restrictions and provides adequate nutrition.

Environment

The environment in which meals are taken is, to some extent, outside the control of the nurse but, at the very least, it should be different from the one in which the patients normally sleep and socialize. There is much, otherwise, that the nurse can do to ensure an environment—regardless of any physical or architectural constraints—that is conducive to mealtimes (Hotaling, 1990). This includes proper seating and tables, pleasant surroundings, for example flowers on the tables and pictures on the wall, a peaceful unhurried mealtime which is free from disturbance by other members of the multidisciplinary team and from unnecessary disturbance by nursing staff. This may require the nurses to reschedule medication rounds

---

Helping the patient to eat and drink

Environment
Conducive to eating and drinking, different from area for sleeping and recreation; pleasantly decorated; quiet; undisturbed by medical, therapeutic and nursing staff (medication rounds); appropriate seating for individual patients—height of tables should accommodate wheelchairs

Choice
A choice of menu should be available; nurses should liaise with other departments to ensure that this is so; patients may require help with choosing appropriate food from menu

Aids
Feeding aids for individuals should be specified in care plans; these should be available on the ward at every mealtime

Assistance
Nurse should be comfortable; only one patient should be fed at a time; patient should not be hurried; trained staff should decide when patient has finished meal; individual dignity should be preserved

Supplements
These should only be given according to locally agreed guidelines

---

Box 10.4

and clinical visits by the geriatric team. Individuals who require or who wish to eat alone should be enabled to do so, provided that adequate supervision is available.

Aids

Helping individuals who have feeding difficulties should be seen as a priority for nursing staff at mealtimes. This may require the provision of a special time for such patients when sufficient staff are available. The necessity of having nursing handovers and staff meal breaks during such times should be questioned and any problems brought to the attention of senior nursing staff so that adequate staff can be provided. The kind of help that is required can range from friendly encouragement to eat to complete assistance with feeding. In many cases specialized cutlery, crockery and non-slip mats may be required, and the best results can often be obtained by consulting the occupational therapist. At the very least, the requirements of individuals should be stated in care plans and nurses should ensure that an adequate supply of such feeding aids is provided to fulfil the needs of all the patients.

Assistance

When assistance with feeding is being given to individuals it is essential that this is done in an unhurried way and in a way which is dignified for the individual (Greenhorn, 1992). The nurses giving assistance should be seated comfortably beside the patient and in such a way that feeding can take place without spillage and aspiration of food. Protective clothing for the patient, such as bibs, should only be used if it is absolutely necessary. Nurses should ensure that hygiene standards are maintained by having clean hands and trying not to become involved in nursing tasks with other patients while they are involved with feeding.

Swallowing

Some elderly people, particularly following cerebrovascular accident but also in cases of multiple sclerosis
and motor neurone disease, will have difficulty in
swallowing. It may be dangerous for nurses to proceed
with feeding such patients without the advice of a
speech therapist. If soft diets are required then the
dietitian's advice should be sought in order that a
nutritionally adequate diet can be provided. All such
aspects of specialist advice and prescriptions should
be recorded in the nursing care plans.

Supplements

Supplements should only be used as prescribed or as
replacements for meals according to locally agreed
standards. For example, it may be specified by the
dietitian that a supplement can be given for meals
missed over a 24-hour period after which, if the
problem of missing meals persists, the dietitian should
be consulted. Supplements are expensive, and it may
be counter-productive for individuals to administer
them inappropriately over a prolonged period.

Social and Cultural Factors

In assessing the individual elderly person from the
nutritional point of view, and subsequently helping
the person to eat and drink, it is necessary for the
nurse to take into account aspects of the person's social
and cultural background. Within one culture people
have many different habits in relation to food and this
becomes even more apparent between cultures. If an
elderly person is used to praying before a meal or

undergoing an elaborate ritual of cleansing then this should be accommodated. However, there are simpler things, such as going to the toilet, washing of hands and saying grace, which should also not be overlooked.

CONCLUSION

Elderly people have particular problems regarding nutrition. They are at greater risk of developing malnutrition and are more susceptible to the effects of malnutrition. Nurses play a crucial role in the nutrition of elderly people, and this is particularly true in hospital. Much can be learned about nutrition in the initial assessment period of an elderly person to hospital and the single most important indicator of nutritional status is body weight. This can also be followed throughout the course of an admission in order to monitor the nutritional status of an elderly person. Locally agreed standards are required in order for nurses to know when it is appropriate to seek specialist help, via the physician, with nutrition.

The role of the nurse in maintaining an adequate nutritional status is that of helping the individual to eat and drink. This covers many aspects of work connected with the preparation and delivery of food and drink in hospital and brings the nurse into contact with other departments in the hospital and with the multidisciplinary team.

Refusal to eat, which has not been covered in this chapter, poses a particularly difficult problem in the case of an elderly person with dementia. In such cases it is hard to know whether or not the choice to refuse food and drink is deliberate. There are ethical problems when elderly people refuse to eat and drink, and these

will be mentioned in the following chapter on care of
the dying patient.

REFERENCES

Beaton GH (1986) Toward harmonisation of dietary, biochemi-
cal, and clinical assessments: the meanings of nutritional
status and requirements. *Nutrition Reviews* **44**(11): 349–358.

Coates V (1985) *Are They Being Served?* Royal College of
Nursing, London.

Collinsworth R & Boyle K (1989) Nutritional assessment of
the elderly. *Journal of Gerontological Nursing* **15**(12): 17–21.

DHSS (Department of Health and Social Security) (1975)
Nutrition and Health in Old Age. HMSO, London.

Deurenberg P, van der Koog K, Hulsof T & Evers P (1989)
Body mass index as a measure of body fatness in the
elderly. *European Journal of Clinical Nutrition* **43**: 231–236.

Geissler CA & Bates JF (1984) The nutritional effects of tooth
loss. *The American Journal of Clinical Nutrition* **39**: 478–489.

Greenhorn T (1992) Fed up. *Nursing Times* **88**(30): 32–33.

Heaton KW (1990) Dietary fibre. *British Medical Journal* **300**:
1479–1480.

Hotaling DL (1990) Adapting the mealtime environment.
Dysphagia **5**: 77–83.

Kositzke JA (1990) A question of balance: dehydration in
the elderly: *Journal of Gerontological Nursing* **16**(5): 4–11.

Kwok T & Whitelaw MN (1991) The use of armspan in
nutritional assessment of the elderly. *Journal of the American
Geriatrics Society* **39**: 492–496.

Lehmann AB (1989) Review: undernutrition in elderly people.
Age & Ageing **18**: 339–353.

Rajcevich K & Wakefield B (1991) Altered nutrition: less than
body requirements. In Maas M, Buckwalter KC & Hardy
M (eds) *Nursing Diagnoses and Interventions for the Elderly.*
Addison Wesley, Redwood City, pp. 97–105.

Simopolous AP (1985) The health implications of overweight
and obesity. *Nutrition Review* **43**(2): 33–40.

Storrs AMF (1985) *Geriatric Nursing* 3rd Edition. Baillière
Tindall, London.

Watson R (1989) Care of the mouth. *Nursing* **3**(44): 20–24.

Watson R (1990) Feeding patients who are demented. *Nursing Standard* **4**(44): 28–31.

BIBLIOGRAPHY

Arras JD (1988) The severely demented, minimally functional patient: an ethical analysis. *Journal of the American Geriatric Society* **36**: 938–944.

A case study approach to end-of-life issues in demented patients.

Chenitz WC (1991) Alcoholism in the elderly. In Chenitz WC, Stone JT & Salisbury SA (eds) *Clinical Gerontological Nursing*. WB Saunders, Philadelphia, pp. 507–520.

Looks at all aspects of alcohol abuse in the elderly.

Damon L (1988) Nutritional considerations. In Matteson MA & McConnel ES (eds) *Gerontological Nursing Concepts and Practice*. WB Saunders, Philadelphia, pp. 623–648.

A very comprehensive and detailed chapter covering physiological, economical and pharmacological factors.

Eaton M, Mitchell-Bonair IL & Friedman E (1986) The effect of touch on nutritional intake of chronic organic brain syndrome patients. *Journal of Gerontology* **41**(5): 611–616.

The importance of touch as a means of communication is investigated here with beneficial results.

Kunkel ME (1991) Nutrition and Ageing. In Baines EM (ed.) *Perspectives on Gerontological Nursing*. Sage, Newbury Park, pp. 323–338.

A concise up-to-date chapter on the nutritional problems of the elderly—both physiological and psychosocial.

Lennard-Jones JE (1992) *A Positive Approach to Nutrition as Treatment*. King's Fund, London.

A recent report from this very influential body, covering all aspects of nutrition in hospital.

Maas MT & Tandy L (1991) Impaired swallowing. In Maas MT, Buckwalter KC & Hardy M (eds) *Nursing Diagnoses and Interventions for the Elderly*. Addison Wesley, Redwood City, pp. 106–116.

A very good chapter on this particular problem.

National Academy of Sciences (1989) National Academy of Sciences Report on Diet and Health: *Nutrition Reviews* **47**(5): 142–149.

A very good summary of the most recent dietary advice from North America.

Chapter 11
Care of the Dying

For the nurse, the opportunity to be with the dying person should be considered one of the greatest privileges in life. It is inevitable, in the course of caring for elderly people, that a high number of them will die. About 30% of elderly patients die within the first fortnight of admission to an assessment ward, and there are regular deaths in continuing-care settings (Storrs, 1985; Corrado, 1989). Often many deaths will take place within a relatively short period of time, during epidemics of, for example, influenza. Nurses working in such environments, therefore, quickly become accustomed to dealing with death and dying and there is a considerable amount of good practice which can be shared between nurses working in care of the elderly.

The hospice movement has been at the forefront of promoting pain-free death with dignity but the needs of elderly people who are dying, at home or in hospital, are no less than those of terminally ill patients. The majority of deaths continue to occur in hospital, and this chapter will focus on this environment.

One of the few things which the nurse has in common with every person who requires care is that they will both die. In approaching the subject and, indeed, in approaching the dying person each nurse confronts the issue of their own mortality. Nurses form very intimate relationships with the dying patients in their care and it is necessary, in a way which is not necessary for many other caring professionals, for them to take time to come to terms with death. The nurse will be obliged to have a clear view of what death means for the individual, for friends and for family and, based on this view, should be enabled to deliver care to the dying person which is commensurate with comfort and dignity (Hockley, 1989; Hurtig & Stewin, 1990).

It is not the purpose of a textbook of this nature, however, to discuss the ways in which nurses encounter death and dying. Rather, the aim here is to raise some practical issues about the end of life and the role of the nurse in helping patients who are dying in care of the elderly settings.

DEATH WITH DIGNITY

To die with dignity means that one has been treated with respect. Such respect can be basic, in other words that one has been treated in a way which is humane and which would be afforded to all human beings, but it can also mean that personal wishes have been respected and that every reasonable effort has been made to comply with these.

It is impossible to look at the issue of death with dignity without considering decisions about the end of life. Such decisions are not the exclusive realm of any one person or professional group but include the dying person, the relatives and those caring for the person. The subject of euthanasia is commonly raised in this respect, but it will not be given separate treatment in this chapter. It continues to be illegal in the United Kingdom. A fuller consideration of euthanasia will be given in the chapter on *Issues in Caring for Older People* (Chapter 12).

Knowledge of Dying

Some elderly people will have expressed their wishes about dying and others, when confronted with the possibility of death, will have clear ideas about the extent to which they wish their underlying condition to be treated and how much they simply wish to be kept comfortable and allowed to die. This assumes some knowledge on the part of the elderly person about their impending death but difficulties arise, in this respect, under two particular circumstances. First, when an elderly person does not know that they are dying and has not been informed or does not wish to know and, second, when they are incapable of understanding that death is imminent. The latter is particularly true of elderly people with dementia.

When an elderly person has expressed clear wishes about the extent to which they wish to be treated and, basically, to be kept alive for as long as possible or allowed to die, then the wishes of the individual are normally paramount provided that the means for sustaining life are not considered to be extraordinary. It is not possible to present hard and fast rules but it would, for example, be considered extraordinary to perform a coronary artery by-pass operation on an elderly person with advanced cerebrovascular disease. Such decisions are, in any case, outside the scope of responsibility of the nurse. However, the nurse can ascertain what the wishes of an individual are and plays a very important role in making sure that the available choices and medical decisions are explained to the elderly person and to families.

As described above, difficulties arise when wishes have not been expressed by an elderly person, as often happens in cases of dementia. In such cases it is necessary to liaise with relatives, where these are available, and to have adequate consultation between members of the medical and nursing staff.

Informing Patients

One of the issues which arises in relation to death with dignity is that of whether or not an elderly person should always be told when they are dying. Very few elderly people will not have considered the possibility of their own death, and it is not uncommon for elderly people to have made elaborate arrangements for their own funerals and the distribution of their belongings after death by means of a will. However, it must not be assumed that they know when death is imminent and that they necessarily wish to know that the end is near.

In common with the decision about whether or not to sustain life, it is not possible to state clearly whether or not an elderly person should always be informed. When an elderly person is entering the terminal states of their illness it is certainly the responsibility of the nurse to ascertain the extent to which they understand their condition and also their desire to have more knowledge. Such information can be gathered in conversation with the person and by consulting relatives. There can be very few circumstances in which close relatives should not be informed, and it is possible to say, without doubt, that in circumstances where the individual has expressed a wish to know that they are dying the truth should always be told. Another axiom is that, unless local policies dictate otherwise, there is no good reason why the relatives and the individual elderly person should not be informed about the possibility of imminent death by a member of the nursing staff.

Acceptance of Death

When a person is told that they are going to die, the acceptance of this fact is not usually immediate. The states in acceptance of death are shown in Box 11.1 (Thornton, 1991). Commonly, people will go through

---

Stages in acceptance of death

Denial or disbelief
Behave as if it is not true, continue to make plans for the future, refuse to discuss treatment with medical or nursing staff

Anger
Anger at the fact that death is imminent and this may be expressed to medical and nursing staff or towards ministers of religion

Bargaining
Seek second opinion, undertake activities which they think will give them more time

Depression
The truth about the prognosis gradually dawns and the person begins to accept it

Acceptance
The person accepts the diagnosis and begins to cooperate in making decisions about pain control and discussing practical aspects about their terminal care

---

Box 11.1

a stage of denial or disbelief. This denial can also be evident in relatives of the dying person. During this stage it is very hard to make sensible plans about dying and nurses need to be aware of this. It will be difficult, with someone going through denial, to talk to them about their illness, and the person may even behave as if nothing is imminent and carry on making plans for the future which cannot be fulfilled. In caring for the dying person and the relatives of a dying person it is necessary to help them through this stage and not to try to force further information upon them or to attempt to make them accept the inevitable before they are ready. Normally, the initial stage will pass and the dying person may experience a period of anger at the fact they are dying and this may be expressed towards nurses, physicians, family and even against God. Again, this is part of the normal process of accepting death and the dying person needs to be helped through it with honest answers and assurance of practical, realistic help wherever possible.

Bargaining

A period identified as bargaining may follow where the dying person, while accepting the prognosis of imminent death, may try to undertake activities which they think will give them more time. They may seek a second opinion regarding their diagnosis and prognosis and even go away for a period in order to get away from the reality of the fact that they are dying. Sometimes the period of bargaining will be followed by depression as the inevitable begins to dawn and, whether or not depression is present, the person will normally move towards acceptance of their imminent death. Throughout the process of acceptance of death, including all of the stages identified here, it is important for the concept of hope to be kept alive in the dying person. This hope is not unrealistic and does not offer them survival or a miracle cure but engenders the feeling that all is not 'hopeless', that painful symptoms can be controlled, that there is still time to make certain arrangements, that they will not be left alone and that they will, indeed, die with dignity.

NUTRITION IN TERMINALLY DEMENTED PATIENTS

The subject of feeding older people who are in the final stages of a dementing illness is worthy of special consideration and much has been written on it. Frequently it is the case that the elderly person with dementia will not have expressed wishes about how they would like to be treated at the end of life and, given the nature of the condition, it is very difficult to gain an insight into the wishes of the elderly person when they are severely cognitively impaired.

The subject is particularly pertinent to nurses in the United Kingdom and Europe because the treatment of terminally demented patients here, with respect to nutrition, differs markedly from the treatment given in the United States of America. In the United States the possibility of tube feeding is always considered and often implemented. In such cases, in common with the final decision to withhold or continue medical treatment, the decision rests with the physician. In law, the final decision regarding medical treatment similarly lies with the physician in the United Kingdom, as does the final decision about prolonging life by artificial feeding. The decision to artificially feed, however, is rarely implemented in the United Kingdom, and the final decisions about the extent to which a terminally demented elderly person is to be rendered assisted feeding is, in fact, often left to nursing staff.

Refusal to Eat

As discussed in the previous chapter on *Nutrition* in the elderly, the dementing elderly person inevitably requires assistance with feeding, and the terminal stages of dementia are characterized by the complete loss of the ability to feed and often by a complete refusal to feed (Norberg et al, 1980). The question arises as to how this refusal to feed is to be interpreted. Is it really a conscious refusal of food and an expression of the wish to die or is it merely an inevitable consequence of the dementia? There is no answer to this question and no specific guidelines exist, but the end-stages of dementia bring the nurse into the realm of decision making about how much effort should be made to encourage and assist the older person to take food and drink. There would appear to be some consensus that the practice of force feeding is to be avoided and, when assistance becomes force feeding, which is not commensurate with the comfort and dignity of the elderly person and which causes obvious distress, the time has come to accept that feeding should no longer be continued.

NURSING CARE OF THE DYING PERSON

Caring for the dying elderly person is no different from the care of any person who is dying and can be summarized as shown in Box 11.2.

Pain

It is generally accepted that there is no reason for a dying person to experience pain, and the hospice movement has been at the forefront of experimenting and demonstrating how regular analgesia can be administered with only minimal side effects in the terminal stages of an illness. Nurses, and indeed physicians, should overcome any fear or prejudice which they have about the use of opiates in terminal illness. When pain is present it has been shown that the unwanted effects, particularly dependence, are minimal, and doses which are titrated and timed to match the pain being experienced by the dying person are essential to provide comfort. In order to administer the appropriate doses it is necessary for nurses to use some kind of method for assessing the pain being experienced, and a number of tools, such as the visual analogue scales, are available.

Aspects of caring for the dying person

Controlling pain and other symptoms

Maintaining independence for as long as possible

Alleviating isolation, anxiety and fear

Working towards a comfortable, dignified end

Providing support for the patient's family and friends both before and after death

---

Box 11.2

Independence

Independence can be maintained in the dying person by involving them in decision-making about every aspect of their care. The decision, for example, to withhold active medical treatment possibly signals the advent of well-planned and frequent nursing intervention, but this should always be delivered, when possible, in consultation with the dying person. The need for aggressive treatment should always be questioned and in the terminal stages it may even be necessary to question the need for regular positional change if this is not going to be of benefit to the dying person, and especially if it is going to cause distress.

Fear

It is almost inevitable that fear and anxiety will be present to some extent in the dying person and, while there is a natural tendency to wish to give the dying person privacy, this may not be what they wish. At the very least, every effort should be made to facilitate visits by friends and family to the dying person in hospital, and it may even be possible for spouses and close relatives to be accommodated in the hospital in order that they can be close to their husband, wife or parent. If the dying person has an expressed religious preference, then the priest or minister of their religion should be made welcome on the ward and given as much access to the person as required.

Comfort

Physical comfort is paramount in the dying person and much of this will be accomplished by keeping them free of pain as well as being comfortable in the psychological sense. In particular, attention should be paid to care of the mouth, as the dying person will be eating and drinking very little. Some ingenuity is required on the part of nursing staff in providing effective mouth care, but a simple strategy is regular sips of a drink which the dying person likes; if they are unable to drink and swallow, ice cubes or small drops of fluid may suffice. Attention should be paid to any sources of discomfort for the dying person; these may include constipation, breathlessness, pressure areas, personal hygiene and bad odours from wounds or incontinence.

Family

The family and friends of the dying person will also require an element of care. They will want to be assured, at the very least, that the dying relative is not going to be left alone and nursing staff can relieve them and also spend time with them simply talking and providing physical and emotional support. When death is very imminent, it should be possible for a member of the nursing staff to be present to immediately comfort relatives and to explain what is happening. After the person has died then the relatives should be permitted time to stay with the deceased and should not be hurried in any way. Nurses will encounter a great variety of cultural, social and religious responses amongst relatives to the death of a loved one, and the role of the nurse is to help the relatives through the initial stages of the process of mourning. Mourning may follow similar stages to that of accepting death. The initial numbness at the loss of a loved one may yield to a stage of protest at the loss and a great

yearning to have the loved one back again. Once the
loss has been accepted, a period of great apathy and
depression can set in, which is quite normal and may
last for many months or even years. The nurse in
hospital is only involved at the very beginning of this
process, but further help may be available through
voluntary counselling organizations.

After Death

Following death there are a great many practical details
to be attended to, such as certifying the death and
carrying out last offices, according to local procedures.
The need for these details to be explained to the
relatives and any particular wishes which the relatives
may have in respect to last offices, needs to be
ascertained. In some religions, it is the family which
will carry these out or, in some cases, a minister of
the religion to which the family adheres. The nurse
can offer much advice in the immediate period following death, and details such as whether the deceased
will be buried or cremated need to be broached in
order that the appropriate documentation can be
completed by the medical staff. The relatives need to
be assured that the deceased will continue to be treated
with due respect and dignity; this includes liaising
with the undertakers who will ultimately collect the
remains from the hospital mortuary.

CONCLUSION

Nursing older people and caring for the dying person
and relatives of the dying person are very closely
linked. Whatever skills nurses working with elderly

SECTION IV: ISSUES AND TRENDS

Chapter 12
Issues in Caring for Older People

This chapter is going to deal with a number of issues in care of the elderly which run through the whole of this area of nursing. They could apply to any and all of the previous chapters but they have been selected out because they are emerging issues and ones which merit consideration on their own. Their position in this volume, near the end and collectively, should not be taken to indicate that any less importance is attached to any of them than to the more 'mainstream' aspects of caring for elderly people, such as incontinence or nutrition.

The first issue is medication in older people, many aspects of which differ from medication in other age groups. Other issues considered here therefore include abuse of elderly people, which is receiving increasing attention from the media and professional and voluntary bodies. Closely related to abuse is the subject of restraint, which has been researched and written upon by several authors. Consent with elderly people is considered because there are particular problems, both with treatment and research, in dealing with elderly people who are cognitively impaired.

It is generally considered, for legal purposes, that consent by proxy similar to that obtained for children is sufficient with elderly people who cannot take decisions for themselves, but this is questionable.

Sexuality, while it has been covered in recent nursing literature, is still often overlooked in practice. It should be appreciated that many elderly people, sick and well, have the rull range of normal emotional and physical responses of their younger counterparts. Finally, euthanasia, a topic which is regularly aired in the media and which receives increasingly serious attention in professional publications, is considered in isolation from care of the dying.

MEDICATION

Medication in older people requires special attention and the issues raised span the community/hospital interface and the means to improving therapy and compliance are currently the subject of much research and innovation in nursing. The underlying problem with drug therapy in older people is that they have physiological changes whereby the effect of most drugs is increased, including the side-effects (Watson, 1992). Nurses need to be acutely aware of this as they are often in the 'front-line' for identifying problems which may be arising in elderly people from the drugs they are taking, both medically prescribed and self-prescribed. On the whole, elderly people have less fat deposits and body water than younger people. This means that drugs that are either water or fat soluble are increased in concentration in the bloodstream and this potentiates their action. Furthermore, changes in some organs, principally the kidneys, mean that the body is less able to excrete drugs and their metabolic products.

Problems

The practical outcome of the these age-associated changes is that smaller doses of drugs tend to be prescribed for elderly people. However, it is also the case that, as elderly people often have more than one condition, and several of these may require drug therapy, they are taking many different drugs. This phenomenon of *polypharmacy* can lead to problems through drug interactions and potentiation of the effects of some drugs. As an example, a patient who is suffering from a degree of heart failure and oedema may be prescribed digoxin and a diuretic. The diuretic may lead to reduced blood volume and potentiation of the effects of digoxin, including digoxin toxicity. The same patient may be depressed and therefore prescribed an anti-depressant. The side-effect of some anti-depressants is to cause urinary retention; obviously this will cause discomfort for an elderly person who is also taking a diuretic which increases production of urine. If the patient cannot sleep then a sedative may be prescribed and it may lead to the development of incontinence, particularly at night.

It may appear as if older people cannot win where drugs are concerned but that need not be the case. Regular assessment can establish if every drug is required. It should be a policy to stop the prescription of certain drugs when they are no longer required, and the question on every nurse's mind regarding drugs in older people should be 'Is it really necessary?' They should be willing and able to liaise with general practitioners over this.

Administration and Compliance

Moving away from the specifically physiological and pharmacological problems of drug therapy in older people, other problems of administration quickly become apparent, particularly in the community. It is quite useful to compare the situation in the community with the situation in hospital, which are the two main environments where nurses are involved with drugs. In hospital it is the nurse's responsibility to administer prescribed medication. The drugs are hospital property, the regimen is laid down on the prescription sheet by the doctor and, with only very few exceptions, the nurse is once again very much in control of the situation. Also, it should become apparent very quickly if an elderly person's drug regimen is having undesirable effects and this can be relatively easily corrected. There are a whole host of potential problems which an individual may have in complying with drug therapy which are never highlighted by observing the patient in hospital.

Inevitably, the elderly person is sent home with medication to take, or the district nurse will encounter elderly people with drugs prescribed by their general practitioner. The elderly person may have any of the problems in Box 12.1. It may, in fact, be necessary for a district nurse to visit for the purposes of giving an elderly person their medication and to monitor their condition and reaction to the drugs. On the other hand, there are strategies that can be enacted in order to help elderly people cope better with drug therapy in the community. The process, in fact, begins in hospital where it is possible, after a period of time and in preparation for discharge, to allow patients to self-medicate (Webb et al, 1991). This process requires

---

Problems experienced by the elderly in drug compliance

Confusion

Poor memory

Poor eyesight

Poor grip

Poor understanding of the necessity to comply with the prescribed regime, even if they do not have any of the above problems

---

Box 12.1

somewhere safe for the storage of drugs and also requires monitoring by registered nurses to see how effective it is being with any one individual. In this way, problems can be dealt with and the patient can be discharged with a system of self-medication which really works. There is evidence that this does improve compliance with drug therapy.

In the Community

In the community, the first angle of approach, if an elderly person is having difficulty with drug compliance would be to liaise with a spouse or other close relatives. Of course, their understanding of the need for compliance and their actual ability to help would have to be ascertained before they were left with the task. For the individual there is the possibility of providing them with containers that have tops (non-child proof) that can be easily opened and large labels and clear instructions, and with visual *aide-mémoires* which show examples of the tablets to be taken, for example sellotaped on to a piece of card, and with the times clearly written beside them. It is, of course, possible to be more flexible in the patient's home; if a drug is to be taken three times a day then the first dose does not have to be taken at 06.00 hours, for example. It is really up to the imagination of the district nurse as to how much independence, with safety, an elderly person at home can achieve with their medication.

Self-prescribed Medication

At home another aspect of medication that does not arise in hospital is 'self-prescribed' medication. This may be quite harmless but can, on occasions, be detrimental or dangerous. For example, an over-the-counter antacid may interfere with the uptake of many drugs, including antibiotics, from the gastrointestinal tract. Of a more serious nature is the fact that many over-the-counter cold remedies and analgesic remedies contain paracetamol; if a patient has also been prescribed paracetamol then they may be at risk of taking an inadvertent overdose of paracetamol, which can be fatal. The district nurse can give advice to patients and relatives on how to store drugs safely. This particularly applies to controlled drugs and especially if there are children around who may be able to get their hands on them.

Keeping Medicines

Elderly people are notorious for storing up large quantities of medicine in their homes. This is achieved by buying over-the-counter preparations and also by keeping prescribed drugs which they have not used. The latter situation can arise because they often do not finish a course of drugs, preferring to stop taking them when they feel better, rather than when the condition has been treated. This is especially true of antibiotics and raises its own problems. The district nurse is in an ideal situation to discourage older people from doing this but must bear in mind that all drugs, including prescribed and controlled drugs which a patient has at home, are the property of the patient and the nurse has no mandate to remove or destroy the drugs without permission from the patient or his/her family. In the case of a deceased person, it is wise to dispose of any controlled drugs which may be left. The legal consequences of the drugs falling into the wrong hands could be explained to the family and the drugs destroyed in the presence of a witness.

The pharmaceutical services have a key role to play in ensuring that patients at home take their medicines safely and comply with the prescribed regimens. Nurses should also view the pharmacist, either in the hospital or in the community, as a resource for information and guidance. The Scottish Home and Health Department (SHHD, 1989) commissioned a study into the issue of pharmaceutical services for older people, and among the recommendations of the report were those shown in Box 12.2.

ABUSE OF ELDERLY PEOPLE

Abuse is something which, by its very nature, happens to people who are in positions where they are physically, financially and emotionally dependent upon others. Thus, children are abused within families,

---

Recommendations for pharmacy services for the elderly

Self-medication programmes for selected patients should be initiated or developed

Health boards should make more funding available for hospital pharmacists to undertake a follow-up visit for those patients discharged from hospital who are likely to experience difficulties with medication

Close communication should occur with community pharmacists, general practitioners and community nurses in order to alleviate any problems

Educational programmes should be initiated for the carers of older people as well as for older people themselves

Closer liaison between pharmacists and prescribers is required in order that patients requiring assistance with medication are identified

---

Box 12.2

wives are abused by their husbands and junior employees are abused by more senior colleagues, as sometimes happens in the armed forces. There are, therefore, certain situations where those who abuse can exercise their powers over others in ways which are unacceptable to the individual who is abused and contrary to the norms of society. Another scenario, which encompasses all of the above situations, is that of the abuse of those who are in care. In this manner children are abused in residential care and, as increasingly comes to light, elderly people are abused both at home and in institutional care. In all of these settings the abuse can take many forms encompassing a whole range of activities from the psychological to the physical. For the above reasons, therefore, it is difficult to arrive at one simple definition of abuse but a useful description is the 'deprivation of quality of life' (Tomlin, 1989).

Research on Abuse

Several bodies have turned their attention to the subject of abuse in the elderly; a working group of the British Geriatric Society found that eight categories of abuse were identifiable. These, which mainly refer to abuse in the community, can be summarized as shown in Box 12.3 (Tomlin, 1989).

Those at Risk

The elderly person who is most at risk of being abused is one who is highly dependent and who also has communication difficulties or fluctuating abilities. This particularly applies to the elderly people with Parkinson's disease and dementia. Victims are also, classically, over 75 years of age and female. Abuse at home typically takes place when the burden of care becomes too great for the person administering care to cope with the demands made upon them. The predisposing factors include a great dependence upon one carer, which may engender a feeling of bitterness towards other members of the family who should be sharing the burden. There may be a causative or resulting breakdown in communication within a family, accompanied by poor communication with the dependant. The carer who abuses may have undergone a change in lifestyle from, for example, an active to a non-existent social life in

Categories of abuse

Assault
Force-feeding, shaking and slapping

Deprivation of nutrition
Failing to provide sufficient food and drink either as a punishment or through wilful or 'forgetful' neglect

Administration of inappropriate drugs or deprivation of prescribed drugs
Over-sedation or withholding drugs in order to precipitate a crisis

Emotional and verbal abuse
Intimidation, humiliation, shouting, swearing and emotional blackmail

Sexual abuse
Of low incidence with the elderly, but can involve any members of a family

Deprivation of help in performing activities of daily living
Failure to provide articles such as spectacles, hearing aids and appropriate clothing

Involuntary isolation and confinement
Locking in rooms or preventing from seeing friends and visitors

Financial abuse
Withholding money or refusing to spend money on dependants who have signed over their pensions

Box 12.3

order to accommodate caring for the dependant, and there may also be an element of role reversal whereby the carer, typically male, may now find himself having to carry out a series of unfamiliar domestic chores.

Indicators of Abuse

There are indicators of abuse in elderly people which have been classified as being either physical or social and emotional by Age Concern (1992). The former category includes a history of unexplained falls and minor injuries in an individual. Other injuries include multiple small bruises, described as 'pepperpot', on the chest or bruising in well protected areas. An abused person may also have finger marks or burns in unusual places, and a history of alcohol abuse in an elderly person or carer is also an indicator. Those indicators described as social and emotional include the elderly person looking anxious, agitated or withdrawn. The elderly person may be confined to one room of the house and may not be properly dressed or clean. Professionals may have difficulty in gaining access to the elderly person and the carer may insist on always being present at interviews.

It must be said, however, that some elderly people bruise very easily. For this reason, some caution is required in interpreting every bruise or mark on the body of an elderly person and, in some cases, caution is required in making use of reports by individual elderly people of abuse which has been inflicted upon them. Nothing will do the cause of eliminating abuse of elderly people more harm than inaccurate reports of abuse which lead to premature and, in some cases, quite unnecessary investigations. It should always be the case that several indicators of abuse should be present, and that detailed discussion between the professionals involved in any case should take place before action is taken.

Handling Abuse Situations

Several professionals—the general practitioner, the geriatrician, the district nurse, the health visitor, the social worker and the nurse in care of the elderly— may encounter the abuse of elderly people. It should be appreciated that abuse is not an easy subject to broach either with the abused or the abuser. Abused elderly people may be reluctant to admit that they are being abused, not wishing to 'betray' a loved one who has been previously cared for them well. Nevertheless, nurses must report all suspected cases of abuse to their line managers and to the abused person's general practitioner and must ensure that an investigation will take place, including action to protect the abused person, if abuse is confirmed. Accurate records must be kept at all stages as these may be required for legal purposes.

It is considered possible, however, to reduce the incidence of abuse by taking appropriate preventative action. The first step is to educate professionals about the possibility of abuse in elderly people. The elderly person who is being abused can be helped, in the short term, by being removed from the source of the abuse and cared for temporarily in residential care or hospital. A non-judgemental attitude is essential; the objective of nursing care is not see the abuser face criminal charges (although this may sometimes be necessary) or to see the abuser being punished (RCN, 1991). Rather, the interests of the abused should be kept at the forefront and, since abuse has highlighted a crisis, the means to resolving that crisis should be sought. Families in which abuse of an older person is taking place require help and counselling. Education in the role of carer and introduction to local support networks are possibilities which should be considered.

RESTRAINT

Most of the abuse described above happens in the community, in the home of the abused person and none of the aspects of abuse described is ever acceptable or beneficial to the individual concerned. Restraint can also be considered to be a form of abuse but was not considered in the previous section because it is not, in fact, always considered abusive to restrain an elderly person and restraint, where it does happen, usually takes place in institutions. Having said that restraint is not always considered to be abusive, it is necessary to state at the outset to this section that excessive or inappropriate restraint definitely falls within the description of abuse and there is a growing awareness of the seriousness of restraining elderly people in hospital. What, however, constitutes excessive or inappropriate restraint? This issue obviously brings the nurse into the realm of delicate decision making and, fortunately, some guidelines are available.

The objective of restraint in institutions is usually to protect the individual, who may be confused or mentally ill, from coming to harm either by falling or by wandering off to potential danger spots. Restraint, therefore, may be carried out for altruistic reasons. Nevertheless, it must be said that, ultimately, restraint is often for the benefit of busy staff and it is carried out at their convenience (ACE, 1988). The need for restraint should always be questioned and where it has been found to be necessary, for justifiable reasons, the nurse manager should always consider whether or not this indicates the need for the allocation of more staff to that area. Restraint is hard to define precisely but, in order to highlight the subject, it should be noted that, unless confined under the apppropriate section of the Mental Health Act in either England or Scotland or subject to legal restraint, a person has the right to be free in speech and movement despite their physical or mental condition. This does not mean that a nurse is always breaking the law in restraining an elderly person who is at risk of injury but it does mean that, whenever restraint is applied, the nurse should be able to justify why it was necessary and give assurance that it was applied for the minimum possible time.

Scope of Restraint

As the subject has received the attention of different bodies the scope of what might be considered to be restraint has widened to include the factors shown in Box 12.4.

Alternatives to Restraint

There are alternatives to restraint and these normally begin with educating nursing staff about the aspects of their practice which constitute restraint. It helps if the nurses are allowed to then look at their practice and decide for themselves which of these aspects constitutes inappropriate or excessive restraint and to see if they can make changes. Some of the alternatives to restraint involve measures such as reality orientation,

---

Scope of restraint

Physical restraint on movement such as cot-sides, adapted chairs and harnesses

Restraints to circulation within a building, such as sedative drugs, arrangements of furniture, inappropriate use of night clothes during the day and baffle locks

Excessive supervision and observation

Attitudes which infantilize the elderly

Financial methods which make the elderly dependent upon the institution

---

Box 12.4

in order to help the older person who may be confused and alienated to know who the nursing staff are, where the elderly person is and why it is necessary for them to be there. The environment can be controlled such that restraint becomes less necessary, and the attitude and comportment of nursing staff has much to do with this. Staff who conduct themselves in a friendly and reassuring manner to the elderly people in their care will help to reduce restlessness and even aggressive behaviour. Instead of locking doors to keep wandering patients in, they can be taken for a walk and accompanied or even diverted to some other acceptable activity. There are very few occasions when cot-sides are necessary, especially on a long-term basis. They actually increase the danger to the patient and are certainly not commensurate with the dignity of the individual (Gray & Gaskell, 1990). Restraint may be necessary in some circumstances, and when it is required a full assessment of the circumstances should be carried out, the assessment should be recorded, the least restrictive method of restraint should be applied, and a time-limit to the application of the restraint should be set. After withdrawing the restraint, the situation of the individual should be reviewed.

Finally, the attitude of nurses and their managers towards falls in patients, provided that everything possible has been done to minimize the possibility of falls (see Chapter 2), has a part to play. Each fall or case of injury to an elderly person who could have been restrained should not be seen as a tragedy and should not be followed by guilt and blame. A thorough investigation of the circumstances of the fall or injury is required and it may be necessary to introduce some changes to the care of the individual. A fall, however, should not initiate panic such that widespread restraining methods are introduced (Cubbin, 1970). Each case of restraint or injury should be treated individually.

CONSENT

It is a common misconception that once people enter health care they have given up many of their rights, including the right to decide what is best for themselves. This is a falsehood and it is no less true of older people than it is of any other group, even if an elderly person is confused, either acutely or chronically. Obviously, there are cases where individuals are unable to make decisions for themselves and the situations which arise must be dealt with. In children for example, up to the age of consent, it is necessary for a responsible adult, usually the parent, to give consent for hospital treatment and for use of the child in any research work. Parental non-consent can, of course, be overrruled by a court of law, and cases of immediate life-saving procedures where consent is not available generally take place without problem.

Consent to Treatment

An older person of sound mind is capable of making all decisions with regard to treatment and entry into research. Problems only arise when an elderly person is cognitively impaired. In such a condition they are unable to make rational decisions but it is not necessary to obtain consent in order to carry out medical or surgical procedures. It is not unusual for discussion to take place with the relatives of an elderly person with dementia, if the person requires treatment that may be considered extraordinary or radical, but the final decision rests with the physician or surgeon in charge of the case. In the case of nursing care, including the administration of drugs which may be carried out daily without consent for the demented elderly person, this is done in the belief that the elderly person would have wished to have it had they been able to make their own decisions. In any case, there can be no question of a withdrawal of care which would lead to the discomfort and even the premature death of a person with dementia.

Consent to Research

Research, however, on the elderly person with dementia resembles the situation in children. It is not legally and ethically possible to proceed with research which may harm a person without consent from a significant person such as the next of kin or legal guardian. The point has to be faced, however, that such consent may not always be what the elderly person would have wished, and it has been known for such proxy consent to be given for research with demented patients who previously expressed that they would not wish to be involved in such programmes (Warren et al, 1986).

The nurse has a duty, therefore, to protect the rights of the individual elderly person who may not be able to take decisions about research or treatment. This may involve ensuring that they receive treatment which they deserve regardless of their cognitive state or entering into discussion with relatives and medical staff when it is felt that active treatment has continued for long enough. In the realm of research, it is certainly the responsibility of the nurse to ensure that no older person has research, including nursing research, carried out inappropriately or unnecessarily on them.

Ethical Committees

Increasingly, it is the case that difficult decisions are being referred to ethical committees, and it has been common practice for the last 30 years that most health authorities require research proposals to be submitted to the scrutiny of local ethical committees. The *ad hoc* nature of ethical committees is giving way to more structured bodies which, in future, will include more nurses.

SEXUALITY IN OLDER PEOPLE

There is provision in most nursing models and, indeed, in nursing care plans for patients of all ages for the 'expression of sexuality'. The provision usually goes no further, however, and it may be due to considerable confusion and embarrassment amongst nurses that this is the case. It is common myth and misconception that the elderly lose all interest in sex (Parke, 1991). On the contrary, sexual relations between married couples can continue into advanced years and, even in the presence of disease and disability, can be carried on with the imagination and adjustment of both partners. This is a sign of maturity and intimacy between couples and is entirely normal. It has been reported that, where the possibility of conception and the responsibility of raising children have been left behind, renewed interest in sexual relations can take place with couples forming deeper physical and emotional bonds than even they ever thought were possible.

Influence of Ageing

It is the case, nevertheless, that sexual activity does generally decline with age. Intercourse tends to take place less frequently and the incidences of sexual arousal are fewer. Moreover, the incidence of actual sexual dysfunction increases and this is defined by changes in sexual function which individuals find 'unsatisfying, unrewarding or inadequate'.

Approaching sexual matters with individuals, young or old, is not an easy matter for the health-care professions. This is probably the case because sexual relations of couples are an entirely private affair and should not, normally, be discussed with anyone outside the partnership. This does not become any more, or less, the case with older people. Helping patients to 'express sexuality', in any case, does not mean that intimate details have to be requested and recorded in care plans. Married, single and bereaved elderly people all have sexual feelings, and it is not implied that they all require expression through physical sexual gratification. Dressing appropriately and playing appropriate roles can be important aspects of the sexuality of an individual, and it is very much part of the nurse's job to help elderly people in their care to undertake these.

Practical Help

Where married couples are concerned, especially in long-term care, there is no reason why intimacy cannot be allowed and privacy provided in hospital or arrangements made for periods at home, where the health of the individuals allows this. In cases where there are difficulties, such as after a myocardial infarction, practical advice such as the use of nitrates before intercourse can be given. Some drugs, such as antihypertensives, may lead to impotence in males and it may be necessary to seek medical advice in this regard. Obviously, it will not always be possible to resume sexual relations in every situation where this is desired, and nurses should approach this with appropriate sensitivity and provide support for the individual (Jones, 1992).

In all matters relating to sexuality it is not up to the nurse to delve into intimate matters unnecessarily but to form the kind of trusting relationship with the elderly person where they can talk and receive advice and help wherever possible. This is, perhaps, not an area where copious records in the nursing notes are required. Reassurance that sexual feelings in old age are entirely normal and, where difficulties are encountered, that love and intimacy remain possible are mainly what is required.

EUTHANASIA

Euthanasia was raised in the previous chapter but only briefly so, in order that it could be more fully discussed here. The subject is almost always brought into discussions of the care of elderly people and chronically sick and is regularly debated in professional, medical and nursing, journals.

As mentioned in the previous chapter, euthanasia continues to be illegal in the United Kingdom but appears to be gaining increasing acceptance in some countries of the world. This is particularly true of Holland, where active euthanasia is being increasingly practised without prosecution of the physicians involved. Even in the United Kingdom, euthanasia is being practised. There are now, also, a number of organizations which exist to help people to hasten their death through 'assisted suicide'. Despite the fact that the publications produced by these societies are not legally available in the United Kingdom, they are, nevertheless, relatively easy to obtain.

Active and Passive Euthanasia

Euthanasia, strictly speaking, is a 'peaceful and easy death' according to the *Oxford Dictionary*, and passive euthanasia is to be distinguished from active euthanasia, which is really the subject that raises concerns. Assisting peaceful and easy death is an apt description of the work of the hospice movement and also the application of terminal care in general and care of the elderly wards. Passive euthanasia, however, does not include taking steps which will actually deliberately hasten the death of a terminally ill individual.

End-of-life Decisions

When the decision to limit, or withdraw, active treatment such as the administration of antibiotics or intravenous fluids to a terminally ill person is made it is done in the opinion that further treatment would be futile, in other words it would not eventually cure the person of their underlying condition, and it would only serve to prolong suffering. As discussed previously, extraordinary procedures such as radical surgery or life support would not normally be applied to terminally ill patients for whom the benefits would be minimal and outweighed by prolonged suffering. Palliative, pain-relieving surgery would normally be carried out if the patient was able to undergo it and, of course, the full range of analgesics and nursing care would be applied to any patient who was terminally ill.

The Debate

The debate about implementing the practice of active euthanasia is between those who think that it is right, if the individual terminally ill person or the person who has previously outlined the appropriate circumstances, to hasten death and thereby alleviate suffering (Ellis, 1992), and those who do not. The former side of the debate attaches much greater importance to the concept of 'quality of life' than to the concept of the 'sanctity of life'. The sanctity of life ethic, if taken to its extreme can mean that life must be preserved at all costs. However, it is at a less extreme level that this argument, whereby the deliberate hastening of death is seen as being morally wrong, is the argument most commonly used by those who oppose active euthanasia.

Both sides of this debate claim to have the interests of the individual, who may be suffering, at heart. Those who oppose active euthanasia would argue that, based on the work of the hospice movement, it is unnecessary to implement this practice because it is always possible to alleviate suffering. On the other hand, those who favour active euthanasia claim that the individual should have the right to refuse further active and palliative treatment and be enabled, with the help of medical and nursing practitioners, to choose when they want to die. A further argument against the implementation of active euthanasia is that it would be the 'thin edge of the wedge' (Trevelyan, 1992) whereby, even if it were acceptable to introduce active euthanasia with the consent of the terminally ill individual, the situation would rapidly develop whereby the decision would be taken by the medical profession, possibly in consultation with relatives, without consulting the individual. This may be a particular problem in cases of the terminally demented.

In whatever way the debate about active euthanasia is finally settled, it appears that an element of active euthanasia is currently being practised. While the practice remains illegal in the United Kingdom, all nurses should consider their position very carefully from the moral, professional and legal points of view before participating in the practice and being asked to observe it without comment. If, in future, the practice of active euthanasia becomes legal and therefore common and widespread in this country, then a new situation in health care will have developed which will be very distressing for many nurses.

CONCLUSION

The list of issues in care of the elderly has by no means been exhausted in this chapter. The issues raised in this chapter are some of those which are currently topical and, in the future, some of these may be resolved and others will come into focus. Nurses have been, and indeed should be, at the forefront of the debate on all of these issues; they should be seeking to educate themselves on the principles involved and, where satisfactory conclusions have been arrived at by the profession, they should be educating each other and the other members of the multidisciplinary team with which they work in caring for elderly people.

REFERENCES

ACE (Royal College of Nursing Association for the Care of the Elderly) (1988) *Newsletter*, Summer: 8–9.

Age Concern (1992) *Abuse of Elderly People: Guidelines for Action*. Age Concern, London.

Cubbin JK (1970) Mechanical restraints: to use or not to use? *Nursing Times* **66**(24): 752.

Ellis P (1992) An act of love . . . *Nursing Times* **88**(37): 34–35.

Gray CS & Gaskell D (1990) Cot-sides: a continuing hazard for the elderly. *Geriatric Medicine* **20**(2): 21–22.

Jones C (1992) Sex and MI: sexual activity after myocardial infarction. *Nursing Standard* **6**(48): 25–28.

Parke F (1991) Sexuality in later life. *Nursing Times* **87**(50): 40–42.

RCN (Royal College of Nursing) (1991) *Guidelines for Nurses: Abuse and Older People*. RCN, London.

SHHD (Scottish Home and Health Department) (1989) *Pharmaceutical Services for Older People—Practical Guidance.* HMSO, Edinburgh.

Tomlin S (1989) *Abuse of Elderly People: An Unnecessary and Preventable Problem.* British Geriatrics Society, London.

Trevelyan J (1992) . . . Or an admission of failure? *Nursing Times* **88**(37): 36–37.

Warren JW, Sobal J, Tenney JH, Hoopes JM, Damron D, Levenson S, DeForge BR & Muncie HL (1986) Informed consent by proxy: an issue in research with elderly patients. *New England Journal of Medicine* **315**(18): 1124–1128.

Watson R (1992) Drugs and the Elderly. *Practice Nursing,* February: 17–18.

Webb C, Addison C, Holman H, Saklali B & Wagner A (1991) Self-medication for elderly patients. *Nursing Times* **86**(16): 46–49.

BIBLIOGRAPHY

Counsel & Care (1992) *What if They Hurt Themselves.* Counsel & Care, London.

An excellent and comprehensive document on the issue of restraint. It looks at a very wide range of nursing interventions which may be considered to be restraining.

Davies P (1992) Elderly and baffles. *Nursing Standard* **6**(21): 49.

The author discusses the pros and cons of using baffle locks with elderly demented patients.

McCarthy DG & Moraczewski AS (1981) *Moral Responsibility in Prolonging Life Decisions.* Pope John Centre, St. Loius.

A very comprehensive look at the subject from the Catholic Christian perspective.

Royal College of Nursing (1987) *Focus on Restraint.* RCN, London.

One of the best documents, including guidelines for nursing staff, which is available.

Scottish Action on Dementia (1992) *Consent to Treatment and Consent to Research.* SAD, Edinburgh

Two very good discussions on the involvement of patients with dementia in medical research and the related area of consent to treatment.

Steinke EE (1991) Sexuality in Ageing. In Baines EM (ed.) *Perspectives on Gerontological Nursing.* Sage, Newbury Park, pp. 78–93.

Concise look at attitudes towards this subject and also to dysfunction in the elderly.

Strumpf NE, Evans LK & Schwartz D (1991) Physical restraint of the elderly. In Chenitz WC, Stone JT & Salisbury SA (eds) *Clinical Gerontological Nursing.* WB Saunders, Philadelphia, pp. 329–344.

Well-known authors on the subject look at the implication of restraint in the clinical setting.

Watson R (1990) Research on the elderly. *Nursing Times* **86**(16): 43–45.

Considers the ethical issues surrounding research on elderly people and looks at research strategies for overcoming problems.

Watson R & Brunton M (1990) Restrain yourself. *Nursing the Elderly* **2**(5): 20–21.

A report showing that it is possible to drastically reduce the use of cot-sides and to maintain safety.

Chapter 13
Care of The Elderly in the Future

The future of care of the elderly is, of course, impossible to predict. Most of what follows is speculative, it picks up on some of the issues raised in the first chapter, and is based on current demographic and social trends. We can be sure, and the figures exist to support this, that the proportion of elderly people in society will increase. The fall in the birth rate, which is very much a problem in many European countries, will take many years to overcome in terms of the number of young people entering the workforce. This problem is already apparent and is probably going to become more acute. There will be a much smaller number of working people supporting an ageing, and increasingly frail, society.

ECONOMIC CONSEQUENCES OF DEMOGRAPHIC CHANGE

The effect of demographic change is twofold. First, there is an economic effect whereby social-security and health-care systems will find it difficult to make adequate provision for the number of people requiring care. This may necessitate higher taxation so that less people pay more in order for social care to be possible. Alternatively, and this is happening in the United Kingdom, the very nature of the health and social services is changing, with increasing moves towards efficiency and more economical ways of caring. This particularly applies to elderly people in the community. It is, indeed, questionable whether the community will be able to support the projected numbers of frail elderly people. The extended family, where the older person would be closely involved with the family in bringing up children and, thereafter, looked after in their declining years, is no longer a feature of our society. Many factors, including greater mobility of the workforce and divorce, may have contributed to this, but it is certainly the case that elderly people who retire in the area where they worked and reared their family, are increasingly unlikely to be living near their families. Whether there will be sufficient provision for the frail elderly who require hospital care in the future remains to be seen, but the levels of dependency amongst elderly people with dementia are demonstrably high and the numbers of such elderly people continues to increase.

EMPLOYMENT OF NURSES

The second effect of the demographic effect is a shortage of young people entering the caring professions. Nursing is still a predominantly female profession, but the number of men entering is increasing. This is a pattern which will probably continue but there is a distinct possibility that, in future, there may be difficulties in finding enough nursing staff to work with elderly people.

INCREASING BURDEN OF CARE

The combined effect of demographic changes and reorganization of health care, with an emphasis on community care, is already being witnessed in that hospital wards which care for elderly people are becoming occupied with increasingly frail patients and there is a concomitant increase in the nursing workload. Unless positive steps are taken, this situation cannot continue for much longer without the possibility of a decline in the quality of care delivered to elderly people.

EDUCATION

While the trends, which all appear to be continuing in future, can be lamented, there is a need for sound policies and even better nursing practice in the future. Initially, the nursing profession needs to recruit sufficient people who have a desire and an aptitude for working with elderly people. If such an aptitude is present then it must be nourished with good nursing education in the care of elderly people. Naturally, many nurses want to work in other specialities, particularly in the acute areas of nursing, and it would be wrong to encourage nurses to work with older people if their hearts lay elsewhere. The responsibility of attracting the right nurses in to working with elderly people largely lies with those in nursing education. The dynamic nature of the subject needs to be presented: it is an increasingly important subject, the proportion of elderly people is increasing, the number of frail elderly people is increasing, a greater proportion of the health-care budget is going in this direction. So do the kind of qualities which are required for the job: patience, perseverance, high standards of care and the ability to work closely with other members of the multidisciplinary team.

Role Models

One of the best forms of education is that of example. In this light, it is the responsibility of all nurses who have chosen a career in care of the elderly to promote a positive image of working with older people. This should not just be done generally but should also be done specifically with the students and less experienced colleagues who work with them. The advent of Project 2000, with the supernumerary status of students, and the related increase in the use of preceptors offers an excellent opportunity for the development of good role models in this area of nursing.

RESEARCH

There is already a large body of research work on the study of ageing and in the nursing care of elderly people. The education of nurses in care of the elderly needs to be based on this research in order to demonstrate that improvements in the care of specific problems of individual elderly people in such areas as pressure sores, incontinence, cognitive function, nutrition and terminal care are possible. Furthermore, the need for further research in these and other areas should be highlighted as a means to attracting nurses with research skills into working with older people.

Gerontological Research

The science of gerontology continues to make advances on a multidisciplinary front. The work involves physicians, biologists, psychologists, sociologists, other scientists and, increasingly, nurses in the study of the ageing process. New knowledge will be gained in the years ahead and one of the problems which is being most intensively studied is dementia. One underlying question remains to be answered and that is whether or not dementia, such as that caused by Alzheimer's disease, is really a disease or just an exaggeration or acceleration of the normal ageing process. On the medical front, the possibility of curing dementia may become a reality but, in the meantime, there is a great deal to be learned about caring appropriately for elderly people with cognitive decline. Nursing research is increasingly turning its attention in this direction and will continue to do so. Important areas for nursing research are the assessment of problems in demented patients and the development of appropriate intervention. Such problems as feeding, wandering, aggression and cognitive decline all merit further attention.

SPECIALIZED UNITS

More specialized units staffed by more specialized nurses may become increasingly common. Already, it appears that there are advantages in housing demented patients together and concentrating on the kind of care which they require. However, both general nurses and psychiatric nurses are involved in the care of elderly people and, as mentioned previously, plans have been made to provide social and nursing care under one roof, with patients progressing through a system of care as their needs increase. Perhaps there is room in future for a qualified generic care worker with an educational background in gerontology and training in both the nursing and social aspects of care.

RETIREMENT

At another level, the future may hold some changes for the older person generally. The declining workforce due to demographic changes may be the necessitating factor. Retirement at 60–65 years of age is very much the norm in the West. Retirement can be viewed as either a blessing or a curse. For some people it is a time of great opportunity, while for others it is a time when they feel that they have been shelved and rejected by society. In some developing countries, retirement is actually a luxury which few can afford, and it is the case that in some African countries over 90% of men of pensionable age (over 65 years) are still working—they cannot afford to stop. Contrast this with Europe, where less than 10% of men of pensionable age are still working.

What may be required, in the West, is a more flexible attitude towards retirement and one which allows those who are still able to support themselves and contribute financially to their economies to do so. Research into working abilities with age has shown that, again contrary to popular opinion, older workers are easily trained to take on new jobs and are, on the whole, a more reliable sector of the workforce than their younger counterparts. With the economic effects of the ageing population described earlier, it may be necessary to deliberately recruit more older workers, leaving the freedom to retire if necessary, into industry in order to provide the resources needed for the greater requirement for health and social care. This could have positive benefits for the elderly people in two ways. It could give them a greater sense of worth in that they are contributing to the economy of the country and, reciprocally, it could lead to a greater respect for older people from the younger members of the workforce.

For those older people who are going into retirement there is a growing awareness that some preparation is necessary. Increasingly, companies are taking this into account and are running their own schemes for the older members of their workforce. It can be quite traumatic for some people to find themselves faced with apparently endless hours of leisure. Despite the fact that they may have been contemplating this with enjoyment, the reality is often very different from their expectations. Suddenly, they are separated from their workmates and, not unnaturally, from many old friends; the leisure which has been thrust upon them may soon be converted into boredom, and depression can follow. For these reasons, it is sometimes appropriate for people to gradually withdraw from work though a gradual reduction in working hours in order that they can 'acclimatize' to the new situation and find new interests and different ways of managing their time at home. In this way, the trauma of eventual transition into full retirement is lessened.

HEALTH EDUCATION

Health education is a subject which is now commonly brought up in relation to elderly people. Certainly it is possible to advise elderly people in more healthy lifestyles and such obvious steps as stopping smoking, eating less fat and taking more exercise are common-place. It is very hard, nevertheless, to evaluate the effectiveness of health education, and the focus of health education, for healthy ageing, should probably be on the young. The British Government's White Paper *The Health of the Nation* is one initiative which aims to promote more healthy lifestyles across all of the age groups of the population. The habits which we develop in our lifetime are the habits which we often take into old age. Allowing for a number of diseases which adversely affect health in later years, it is surely the case that many elderly people have not had the opportunity to develop interests, hobbies and good health habits in their youth. Many young people do not think ahead to their old age but, as lifespan increases and more people reach advanced years the need for education about old age should begin earlier in life. This will not only help the younger generation to appreciate and care for their elders as years are added to their lives, it will help them, in their turn, to add life to their own advanced years.

BIBLIOGRAPHY

George M (1992) The health of the nation. *Nursing Standard* **6**(44): 18–19.

This article looks at the scope and possible implications of the UK Government's White Paper of the same name.

Gray JAM & Blair P (1990) *Your Health in Retirement*. Age Concern, London.

A book written by a physician and a health journalist which looks at some of the ways in which older people can prepare for retirement and maintain their health in retirement.

Masson PR (1990) Long-term macroeconomic effects of ageing populations. *Finance and Development* **27**(2): 6–9.

Written from the economic perspective, this article looks at the worldwide implications of projected demographic changes.

International Labour Organization (1988) Older workers: too young to be dumped. *ILO Information* **24**(5): 1.

International Labour Organization (1991) The elderly; an intolerable burden? *ILO Information* **19**(3): 1.

International Labour Organization (1990) Wanted: older workers. *ILO Information* **26**(1): 7.

International Labour Organization (1990) No retirement for ageing poor. *ILO Information* **26**(4): 4.

International Labour Organization (1991) An active future for older workers. *ILO Information* **28**(1): 4.

All of the above reports from this United Nations specialist body are worth reading. They contain much useful demographic information but also cast a light on the economic importance of older people, not just in the developing world, where they are often unable to retire, but in the developed world where their experience and services may be increasingly required.

Zedlewski SR & McBride TD (1992) The changing profile of the elderly: effects on future long-term care needs and financing. *The Millbank Quarterly* **70**(2): 247–276.

Based mainly on computer predictions, this lengthy article looks at the demographic changes in the United States of America and their economic implications for health and social care.

Appendix: Useful Organizations

Age Concern England
Bernard Sunley House
60 Pitcairn Road
Mitcham
Surrey CR4 3LL

Alzheimer's Disease Society
158–160 Balham High Road
London SW12 9BN

British Association of the Hard of Hearing
7–11 Armstrong Road
London W3 7JL

Brittle Bone Society
Unit 4, Block 20
Carlunie Road
Dunsinane Estate
Dundee DD2 3QT

Carers' National Association
29 Chilworth Mews
London W2 3RG

Chest, Heart and Stroke Association
Tavistock House North
Tavistock Square
London WC1H 9JE

Crossroads (Association of Crossroads Care Attendant Schemes)
10 Regent Place
Rugby
Warwickshire CV21 2PN

CRUSE—Bereavement Care
126 Sheen Road
Richmond
Surrey TW9 1UR

Depressives Association
PO Box 5
Castletown
Portland
Dorset DT5 1BQ

Dial UK (Disablement Information Advice Line)
117 High Street
Clay Cross
Chesterfield
Derbyshire S45 9DZ
Tel. 0246 250 055

Disabled Living Foundation
380–384 Harrow Road
London W9 2HU

Help the Aged
16–18 St James's Walk
London EC1R OBE

Parkinson's Disease Society
36 Portland Place
London W1N 3DG

Royal National Institute for the Blind
224 Great Portland Place
London W1N 6AA

Scottish Action on Dementia
8 Hill Street
Edinburgh EH2 3JZ

Index